Science of Circadian Rhythms

Editor

PHYLLIS C. ZEE

SLEEP MEDICINE CLINICS

www.sleep.theclinics.com

Consulting Editor
TEOFILO LEE-CHIONG Jr

December 2015 • Volume 10 • Number 4

ELSEVIER

1600 John F. Kennedy Boulevard • Suite 1800 • Philadelphia, Pennsylvania, 19103-2899

http://www.theclinics.com

SLEEP MEDICINE CLINICS Volume 10, Number 4
December 2015, ISSN 1556-407X, ISBN-13: 978-0-323-40270-5

Editor: Patrick Manley
Developmental Editor: Donald Mumford

Sleep Medicine Clinics (ISSN 1556-407X) is published quarterly by Elsevier Inc., 360 Park Avenue South, New York, NY 10010-1710. Months of issue are March, June, September and December. Business and Editorial Offices: 1600 John F. Kennedy Blvd., Ste. 1800, Philadelphia, PA 19103-2899. Customer Service Office: 3251 Riverport Lane, Maryland Heights, MO 63043. Periodicals postage paid at New York, NY and additional mailing offices. Subscription prices are $195.00 per year (US individuals), $95.00 (US residents), $406.00 (US institutions), $230.00 (Canadian individuals), $235.00 (international individuals), $135.00 (Canadian and international residents) and $452.00 (Canadian and international institutions). Foreign air speed delivery is included in all *Clinics* subscription prices. All prices are subject to change without notice. **POSTMASTER:** Send change of address to *Sleep Medicine Clinics*, Elsevier Health Sciences Division, Subscription Customer Service, 3251 Riverport Lane, Maryland Heights, MO 63043. Customer Service: **Tel: 1-800-654-2452 (U.S. and Canada); 314-447-8871 (outside U.S. and Canada). Fax: 314-447-8029. E-mail: journalscustomerservice-usa@elsevier.com (for print support); journalsonline support-usa@elsevier.com (for online support).**

Reprints. For copies of 100 or more of articles in this publication, please contact the Commercial Reprints Department, Elsevier Inc., 360 Park Avenue South, New York, NY 10010-1710. Tel.: 212-633-3874; Fax: 212-633-3820; E-mail: reprints@elsevier.com.

Sleep Medicine Clinics is covered in *MEDLINE/PubMed (Index Medicus).*

PROGRAM OBJECTIVE

The goal of *Sleep Clinics of North America* is to keep practicing physicians up to date with current clinical practice by providing timely articles reviewing the state of the art in patient care.

TARGET AUDIENCE

All practicing physicians and other healthcare professionals.

LEARNING OBJECTIVES

Upon completion of this activity, participants will be able to:

1. Review the association of circadian rhythm disorders with psychiatric disorders, neurological disorders, and cardiometabolic problems.
2. Discuss the roles that light, melatonin, and vision play in circadian rhythm disorders.
3. Recognize the effects of both genetic factors and environmental factors such as jet lag and shift work disorders on circadian rhythm.

ACCREDITATION

DISCLOSURE OF CONFLICTS OF INTEREST

UNAPPROVED/OFF-LABEL USE DISCLOSURE

TO ENROLL

To enroll in the Sleep Medicines Clinic Continuing Medical Education program, call customer service at 1-800-654-2452 or sign up online at http://www.theclinics.com/home/cme. The CME program is available to subscribers for an additional annual fee of USD $140.

METHOD OF PARTICIPATION

In order to claim credit, participants must complete the following:

1. Complete enrolment as indicated above.
2. Read the activity.
3. Complete the CME Test and Evaluation. Participants must achieve a score of 70% on the test. All CME Tests and Evaluations must be completed online.

CME INQUIRIES/SPECIAL NEEDS

For all CME inquiries or special needs, please contact elsevierCME@elsevier.com.

SLEEP MEDICINE CLINICS

THE CLINICS ARE AVAILABLE ONLINE!
Access your subscription at:
www.theclinics.com

Contributors

CONSULTING EDITOR

TEOFILO LEE-CHIONG Jr, MD
Professor of Medicine, National Jewish Health;
Professor of Medicine, School of Medicine,
University of Colorado Denver, Denver,
Colorado; Chief Medical Liaison, Philips
Respironics, Pennsylvania

EDITOR

PHYLLIS C. ZEE, MD, PhD
Director, Sleep Disorders Center,
Northwestern Medicine; Director, Center for
Circadian and Sleep Medicine; Benjamin and
Virginia Boshes Professor, Department of
Neurology, Northwestern University Feinberg
School of Medicine, Chicago, Illinois

AUTHORS

SABRA M. ABBOTT, MD, PhD
Assistant Professor, Department of Neurology,
Center for Circadian and Sleep Medicine,
Feinberg School of Medicine, Northwestern
University, Chicago, Illinois

RAVI ALLADA, MD
Department of Neurobiology, Northwestern
University, Evanston, Illinois

TOMAS S. ANDREANI, BA
Department of Neurobiology, Northwestern
University, Evanston, Illinois

RUTH M. BENCA, MD, PhD
Professor, Department of Psychiatry; Director,
Center for Sleep Medicine and Sleep
Research, University of Wisconsin-Madison,
Madison, Wisconsin

HELEN J. BURGESS, PhD
Professor, Biological Rhythms Research
Laboratory, Department of Behavioral
Sciences, Rush University Medical Center,
Chicago, Illinois

EVAN D. CHINOY, PhD
Research Fellow in Medicine, Division of
Sleep and Circadian Disorders, Departments
of Medicine and Neurology, Brigham and
Women's Hospital; Division of Sleep Medicine,
Harvard Medical School, Boston,
Massachusetts

JEANNE F. DUFFY, MBA, PhD
Associate Professor of Medicine, Division of
Sleep and Circadian Disorders, Departments
of Medicine and Neurology, Brigham and
Women's Hospital; Division of Sleep Medicine,
Harvard Medical School, Boston,
Massachusetts

JONATHAN S. EMENS, MD
Associate Professor, Department of Hospital
and Specialty Medicine, Portland VA Medical
Center; Departments of Psychiatry and
Medicine, Oregon Health and Science
University, Portland, Oregon

DAE-SUNG HWANGBO, PhD
Department of Neurobiology, Northwestern
University, Evanston, Illinois

TAICHI Q. ITOH, PhD
Department of Neurobiology, Northwestern University, Evanston, Illinois

STEPHANIE G. JONES, PhD
Associate Scientist, Department of Psychiatry, Center for Sleep Medicine and Sleep Research, University of Wisconsin-Madison, Madison, Wisconsin

KRISTEN L. KNUTSON, PhD
Assistant Professor, Section of Pulmonary and Critical Care, Department of Medicine, University of Chicago, Chicago, Illinois

STEVEN W. LOCKLEY, PhD
Circadian Physiology Program, Neuroscientist, Division of Sleep and Circadian Disorders, Brigham and Women's Hospital; Associate Professor, Department of Medicine, Harvard Medical School, Boston, Massachusetts; Professor, School of Psychological Sciences, Monash University, Melbourne, Australia

KATHRYN J. REID, PhD
Research Associate Professor, Department of Neurology, Center for Circadian and Sleep Medicine, Feinberg School of Medicine, Northwestern University, Chicago, Illinois

SIRIMON REUTRAKUL, MD
Associate Professor, Division of Endocrinology and Metabolism, Faculty of Medicine Ramathibodi Hospital, Mahidol University, Bangkok, Thailand

ALAN M. ROSENWASSER, PhD
Department of Psychology, School of Biology and Ecology, Graduate School of Biomedical Science and Engineering, University of Maine, Orono, Maine

FRED W. TUREK, PhD
Department of Neurobiology, Center for Sleep and Circadian Biology, Northwestern University, Evanston, Illinois

MAKOTO UCHIYAMA, MD, PhD
Professor and Chair, Department of Psychiatry; Professor of Sleep Medicine, Nihon University School of Medicine, Itabashi, Tokyo, Japan

ALEKSANDAR VIDENOVIC, MD, MSc
Assistant Professor of Neurology, Department of Neurology, Massachusetts General Hospital, Harvard Medical School, Boston, Massachusetts

EVRIM YILDIRIM, PhD
Department of Neurobiology, Northwestern University, Evanston, Illinois

PHYLLIS C. ZEE, MD, PhD
Director, Sleep Disorders Center, Northwestern Medicine; Director, Center for Circadian and Sleep Medicine; Benjamin and Virginia Boshes Professor, Department of Neurology, Northwestern University Feinberg School of Medicine, Chicago, Illinois

KIRSI-MARJA ZITTING, PhD
Research Fellow in Medicine, Division of Sleep and Circadian Disorders, Departments of Medicine and Neurology, Brigham and Women's Hospital; Division of Sleep Medicine, Harvard Medical School, Boston, Massachusetts

Contents

considerations that can influence the treatment of choice. The important features of light treatment, light avoidance, exogenous melatonin, and other melatonin receptor agonists are reviewed, along with some of the practical aspects of light and melatonin treatment.

cycles different from 24 hours. Relatively rare in sighted patients, it may be associated with delayed sleep–wake rhythm disorder or psychiatric disorders. It is more common in totally blind individuals owing to the lack of light information reaching the circadian pacemaker in the hypothalamus. We review the clinical characteristics of patients with N24SWD, discuss the biological mechanisms that may underlie its development, and describe treatment strategies.

Irregular sleep-wake rhythm disorder is a circadian rhythm disorder characterized by multiple bouts of sleep within a 24-hour period. Patients present with symptoms of insomnia, including difficulty either falling or staying asleep, and daytime excessive sleepiness. The disorder is seen in a variety of individuals, ranging from children with neurodevelopmental disorders, to patients with psychiatric disorders, and most commonly in older adults with neurodegenerative disorders. Treatment of irregular sleep-wake rhythm disorder requires a multimodal approach aimed at strengthening circadian synchronizing agents, such as daytime exposure to bright light, and structured social and physical activities. In addition, melatonin may be useful in some patients.

Jet lag and shift work disorder are circadian rhythm sleep-wake disorders resulting from behaviorally altering the sleep-wake schedule in relation to the external environment. Not everyone who experiences trans-meridian travel or performs shift work has a disorder. The prevalence of jet lag disorder is unclear, approximately 5%–10% of shift workers have shift work disorder. Treatment aims to realign the internal circadian clock with the external environment. Behavioral therapies include sleep hygiene and management of the light-dark and sleep schedule. Pharmacologic agents are used to treat insomnia and excessive sleepiness, and melatonin is used to facilitate sleep and circadian realignment.

Preface
Circadian Clocks: Implication for Health and Disease

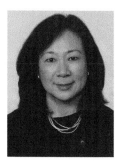

Phyllis C. Zee, MD, PhD
Editor

Recent evidence from animal and human studies indicates that circadian (near 24 hour) rhythms that are regulated by circadian clock genes are intimately involved in the regulation of molecular, cellular, and physiologic functions in central and peripheral tissues. Approximately 20% of all genes are rhythmically expressed, and the circadian system synchronizes biochemical, hormonal, and metabolic processes with feeding behavior, sleep-wake activity, neuropsychiatric function, and daily light-dark cycles. Given the fundamental role of circadian clocks in biological processes, it is perhaps not surprising that disruption of circadian organization results in physiologic aberrations, alterations, and dysfunctions that are relevant for the maintenance of health and development of disease. Aging has been associated with notable changes in sleep and circadian rhythms. For example, in older adults, decreased amplitude of the circadian rest-activity rhythm and greater fragmentation of sleep have been demonstrated to correlate with and predict poor physical and mental health, as well as neuropsychiatric, cardiometabolic, and neurodegenerative disorders. Indeed, the strength and timing of endogenous circadian rhythms and their proper alignment with the external environment are essential for the health of all organisms. As discussed in this issue, the impact of circadian dysfunction and misalignment goes way beyond the circadian sleep-wake disorders, but should be considered in the expression and development of neurologic, psychiatric, metabolic, and cardiovascular disorders. The articles in this issue provide an update on the regulation and interactions of circadian clocks on cardio-metabolic and brain health; evaluate the role of circadian rhythms on brain function and the expression and treatment of age-related neurologic and cardiometabolic disorders, recognition, and treatment of circadian rhythm sleep-wake disorders; and discuss the transformative potential of integrating the time domain in medicine for improving health.

Phyllis C. Zee, MD, PhD
Department of Neurology
Northwestern University
Feinberg School of Medicine
710 North Lake Shore Drive
Suite 520
Chicago, IL 60611, USA

E-mail address:
p-zee@northwestern.edu

Sleep Med Clin 10 (2015) xiii
http://dx.doi.org/10.1016/j.jsmc.2015.09.002
1556-407X/15/$ – see front matter © 2015 Published by Elsevier Inc.

Neurobiology of Circadian Rhythm Regulation

Alan M. Rosenwasser, PhD[a],*, Fred W. Turek, PhD[b]

KEYWORDS

- Circadian • Pacemaker • Suprachiasmatic nucleus • Entrainment • Clock genes

KEY POINTS

- The suprachiasmatic nucleus (SCN) of the anterior hypothalamus has been firmly established as the master circadian pacemaker in mammals.
- The SCN circadian pacemaker is synchronized (entrained) by environmental light-dark cycles via photoreceptors and neural pathways distinct from those mediating visual perception.
- The cellular-molecular basis of circadian rhythm generation involves several circadian clock genes expressed not only in the SCN but also throughout the brain and peripheral tissues and organs.
- The SCN serves as a central pacemaker atop a hierarchically organized, anatomically distributed circadian timing system and entrains downstream circadian clocks via neural and neuroendocrine pathways.
- System-wide circadian coordination is necessary for optimal physiologic function and maintenance of physical and mental health.

IDENTIFICATION OF THE SUPRACHIASMATIC NUCLEUS CIRCADIAN PACEMAKER

The initial demonstrations that lesions of the SCN severely disrupt or abolish circadian rhythms in behavioral and endocrine functions were published in the early 1970s.[1,2] Following these initial demonstrations, extensive subsequent research involving lesions, in vivo and in vitro electrophysiology, functional metabolic mapping, fetal tissue transplant, and molecular analyses revealed that the SCN is capable of autonomous, self-sustained circadian rhythmicity at both the single-cell and tissue levels. These now-classic studies are summarized in the published report of a meeting held to evaluate the state of SCN research on the 25th anniversary of its discovery.[3]

SUPRACHIASMATIC NUCLEUS: A NETWORK OF CLOCK CELLS

Studies using a variety of in vitro models, including electrophysiological recording and optical monitoring of SCN cell and tissue cultures, have provided compelling evidence that circadian oscillation is fundamentally a cell-autonomous process, expressed in many, but probably not all, individual SCN neurons.[4–7] Nevertheless, individual SCN clock cells normally interact to produce coherent circadian signals at the tissue (and behavioral) level.[8–10] Despite the capacity of individual SCN neurons for autonomous rhythmicity, recent studies have revealed that neuronal network interactions increase the frequency of rhythmic cells detected in culture, as well as the amplitude of their

[a] Department of Psychology, School of Biology and Ecology, Graduate School of Biomedical Science and Engineering, University of Maine, 5742 Little Hall, Orono, ME 04467, USA; [b] Department of Neurobiology, Center for Sleep and Circadian Biology, Northwestern University, 2205 Tech Drive, Hogan Hall 2-160, Evanston, IL 60208, USA
* Corresponding author.
E-mail address: alanr@maine.edu

Sleep Med Clin 10 (2015) 403–412
http://dx.doi.org/10.1016/j.jsmc.2015.08.003
1556-407X/15/$ – see front matter © 2015 Elsevier Inc. All rights reserved.

oscillation, and contribute to the overall robustness of SCN pacemaker function.[11,12]

Early studies suggested that SCN clock cells could maintain intercellular synchrony in the absence of sodium-dependent action potentials,[13,14] suggesting that gap junctions, glial coupling, calcium-dependent signaling, or local diffusible signals might be responsible for synchronizing the network of clock cells.[15] In contrast, however, more recent studies have found that blocking action potentials in SCN tissue slices or cell cultures can disrupt intercellular phase synchrony,[10] thus reviving interest in the possible synchronizing role of synaptic transmission. Both γ-aminobutyric acid (GABA) and vasoactive intestinal peptide (VIP) neurotransmission, among other signaling mechanisms, have now been implicated in the maintenance of coupling among SCN clock cells, as well as among subpopulations of SCN clock cells.[16,17]

MOLECULAR BASIS OF THE SUPRACHIASMATIC NUCLEUS CIRCADIAN PACEMAKER

A critical role for protein synthesis in the mammalian circadian pacemaker was established in the late 1980s,[18,19] and elucidation of the fundamental molecular genetic oscillatory mechanism began in earnest about 10 years later. The first mammalian circadian clock gene, Clock, was identified in a forward-genetics mutagenesis screen,[20] and this discovery was followed quickly by the identification of several other core molecular clock components, some of which were homologous to previously discovered circadian clock genes in the fruit fly.[21,22] In addition to Clock, other recognized mammalian clock genes include the 3 period (Per) genes (Per1, Per2, Per3), 2 cryptochrome genes (Cry1 and Cry2), Bmal1 (also known as Arntl1 and Mop3), CK1e (Casein kinase 1 epsilon), Rev-erba, and Fxbl3, all of which are expressed in SCN neurons. The specific functions of these various genes within the interlocking molecular feedback loops that generate circadian signals at the cellular level have been reviewed extensively elsewhere, and are not discussed here.

Mutations or deletions of any of these genes produce alterations in circadian phenotype at the behavioral level. The most devastating effects on clock function are seen in Bmal1 knockout mice, which express immediate loss of rhythmicity in the absence of a light-dark cycle.[21,22] In contrast, the original Clock mutation, which codes for a dominant-negative CLOCK protein, dramatically lengthens free-running period and often leads to a gradual loss of rhythmicity under long-term free-running conditions.[21,22] Surprisingly, however, unlike the original Clock mutation, Clock-null (knockout) mice express robust and persisting circadian rhythms, with only a modest shortening of circadian period[23]; it was subsequently found that NPAS2 can substitute for CLOCK as a dimerization partner for BMAL1 within the SCN, thus maintaining circadian pacemaker function.[24] Regarding the Per genes, several distinct mutations have been studied by different laboratories, but in general, Per1 or Per2 disruption shortens circadian period and reduces the robustness of free-running rhythms.[25,26] Similarly, Cry mutant mice also exhibit alterations in the free-running period, whereas Cry1/Cry2 double mutants are rendered arrhythmic.[27,28] In contrast to other clock genes, the circadian clock function of Ck1e was discovered by genetic analysis of a spontaneous single-gene mutation that dramatically shortens free-running period in the hamster, originally called the tau mutation.[29] Cloning of the tau gene revealed its identity as Ck1e, and subsequent transgenic insertion of this allele into mice recapitulated the hamster short-period phenotype, whereas deletion of Ck1e in mice lengthened the circadian period.[30] More recently, mutations of the Fxbl3 gene have been shown to lengthen the free-running period.[31,32] Like Ck1e, Fxbl3 influences circadian period by regulating the posttranslational stability of other clock proteins such as PER and CRY.[33] Of course, in order for the molecular clock to drive circadian rhythmicity in physiology and behavior, clock gene expression must be linked to intracellular signaling pathways regulating neuronal membrane potential, and ultimately, firing rate. Remarkably, recent research demonstrates that ionic events at the cell membrane influence the molecular clock via some of the same intracellular signals that convey clock signals to the membrane, and in some cases, these ionic currents may be necessary for self-sustainment of the molecular clock.[34] Such results—at a minimum—serve to blur the distinction between the core clock mechanisms and the so-called hands of the clock.

In addition to their effects on circadian behavior, some circadian clock gene mutations also affect sleep-wake homeostasis, and several forms of affective behavior, suggesting possible molecular links between the circadian, sleep regulatory, and motivational systems of the brain.[35–37]

FUNCTIONAL ARCHITECTURE OF THE SUPRACHIASMATIC NUCLEUS

Although the SCN was initially characterized as being composed of distinct ventrolateral and dorsomedial subdivisions,[38] this scheme has been recast to include SCN core and shell subnuclei, a concept that may better accommodate species differences in the anatomic distribution of neuropeptides, afferent terminal fields, and gene expression patterns in the SCN.[39] The SCN core is associated with a high concentration of VIP-positive and gastrin-releasing peptide (GRP)–positive neurons, while the shell is associated with the presence of arginine vasopressin–positive neurons. Beyond this basic organization, however, clear species differences have been noted, and it has been argued that the popular distinction between SCN core and shell may be such an extreme oversimplification as to impede understanding of the functional organization of this critical structure.[40,41]

Although the specific functions of chemically defined SCN cell populations are not fully known, VIP and GRP neurons of the SCN core appear to collate afferent signals relevant to pacemaker entrainment, whereas vasopressinergic (or other) neurons of the SCN shell may have the primary responsibility of generation of self-sustaining circadian oscillations.[42] A preeminent role for the SCN core in pacemaker entrainment is supported by findings that major SCN afferent systems converge in the core subnucleus, administration of SCN core peptides such as VIP and GRP can mimic both light-induced phase shifting and *Per* gene expression in the SCN in vivo and in vitro, and light-evoked changes in SCN physiology and gene expression spreads over time from core to shell. Conversely, evidence for a preeminent role of the SCN shell in pacemaking includes findings that the core projects robustly to the shell, but not vice versa, spontaneous circadian rhythmicity in neuronal activity, neuropeptide release, and gene expression is seen more reliably in the shell than in the core, and spontaneous rhythmicity in SCN gene expression seems to flow from the most dorsomedial toward more central-lateral regions over the course of the circadian cycle. On the other hand, the view that SCN core and shell underlie discrete entrainment and pacemaking functions is probably too simplistic, because (1) several arousal-related afferents of limbic and brainstem origin target the SCN shell,[39] (2) in vitro studies have revealed independent free-running rhythmicity in the secretion of core and shell peptides from the same tissue explant,[43] and (3) SCN core and shell can exhibit stable dissociation of rhythmic gene expression in vivo under certain conditions.[44] Furthermore, studies using microlesions indicate that the integrity of the SCN core is essential for the maintenance of high-amplitude behavioral and molecular-level rhythmicity, suggesting that rhythmic signals from the core serve a permissive gatelike role in sustaining oscillatory function in the shell.[42]

LIGHT INPUT TO THE SUPRACHIASMATIC NUCLEUS: THE RETINOHYPOTHALAMIC TRACT

Although stimuli such as temperature, sound, food, and social cues seem to contribute to phase control, the 24-hour environmental light-dark cycle is the primary cue for circadian entrainment in most mammalians (and other vertebrate taxa). A specialized retinal projection system, referred to as the retinohypothalamic tract (RHT), is both necessary and sufficient for photic entrainment of the circadian pacemaker[45,46] (**Fig. 1**). The RHT originates from a distinct subset of retinal ganglion cells, separate from those giving rise to the primary visual pathways,[47] and terminates mainly in the SCN, as well as more sparsely in the anterolateral hypothalamus, subparaventricular zone, and supraoptic region.[48,49] In addition, RHT axon collaterals also project to the thalamic intergeniculate leaflet (IGL), which, as discussed later, is an important component of the circadian system.

Remarkably, retinally degenerate strains of mice, in which nearly all classic photoreceptors (ie, rods and cones) are lost by early adulthood, exhibit normal circadian responses to light.[50] More recently, similar findings have been reported in genetically engineered mice with a total developmental absence of both rods and cones, demonstrating conclusively that circadian light entrainment can be mediated by a novel, non-rod, noncone photoreceptor system.[51] Circadian entrainment in the absence of rods and cones is maintained by a population of intrinsically photosensitive retinal ganglion cells that use the peptide melanopsin as a photopigment.[52,53] Nevertheless, circadian entrainment is maintained in melanopsin knockout mice[54,55] and is only fully abolished when both classical and melanopsin-based photoreception is eliminated demonstrating redundancy in the circadian photoreception system in the retina.[56–58]

RHT terminals release the excitatory amino acid neurotransmitter, glutamate, which acts through both *N*-methyl-D-aspartate (NMDA) and non-NMDA receptors and a variety of intracellular signaling pathways to increase *Per* gene expression. These changes in gene expression, when superimposed on the ongoing circadian transcription-translation cycle, correspond functionally to phase shifts of the circadian oscillator.[59–62] In addition to glutamate, RHT terminals also release 2 identified peptide cotransmitters,

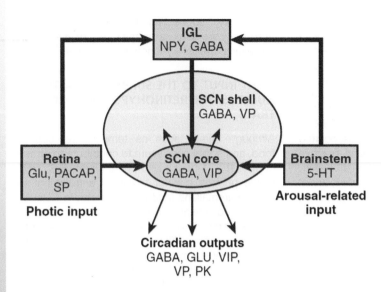

Fig. 1. Overview of functional neuroanatomic pathways in the mammalian circadian system. Major SCN afferent systems originating in the retina and raphe nuclei also target the intergeniculate leaflet (IGL) of the thalamus, which itself projects to the SCN. Retinal projections to the SCN and IGL mediate photic input to the circadian system, whereas raphe projections to the SCN and IGL mediate the effects of certain nonphotic, behavioral state–related signals. Furthermore, raphe-IGL-SCN circuits also modulate and integrate photic and nonphotic signaling to the SCN pacemaker. SCN outputs mainly target the hypothalamus and diencephalon and appear to include both neural efferents and secreted paracrine signals. 5-HT, 5-hydroxytryptamine; GLU, glutamate; NPY, neuropeptide Y; PACAP, pituitary adenyl cyclase–activating peptide; PK, prokineticin; SP, substance P; VP, arginine vasopressin; VIP, vasoactive intestinal polypeptide.

substance P (SP) and pituitary adenyl cyclase–activating peptide (PACAP). SP seems to play an important role in RHT transmission because selective SP antagonists block light-induced phase shifting and immediate-early gene expression in vivo, as well as glutamate receptor–mediated phase shifting in vitro, whereas SP administration can itself induce circadian phase shifts.[63–65] In contrast, PACAP administration has been reported either to antagonize or to mimic the effects of glutamate on circadian phase shifting and *Per* gene expression in vitro, depending on the dose and the circadian phase of administration.[66–68]

OTHER FUNCTIONAL INPUTS TO THE SUPRACHIASMATIC NUCLEUS

An additional major SCN afferent system arises from the IGL, a distinct retinorecipient region of the lateral geniculate complex, intercalated between the dorsal and ventral lateral geniculate nuclei[69–71] (see **Fig. 1**). The projection from the IGL to the SCN is referred to as the geniculohypothalamic tract (GHT), and GHT neurons release both neuropeptide Y and GABA. Retinal signals are conveyed to the IGL in part by axon collaterals of RHT neurons,[72] and GHT and RHT terminal fields are largely coextensive within the SCN core. Thus, the IGL/GHT system provides a secondary, indirect pathway by which light signals can reach the circadian pacemaker. Although the IGL is clearly not necessary for photic entrainment, lesions of the IGL/GHT system result in subtle modifications in the photic control of circadian phase and period.[70,71] Furthermore, the IGL may have a significant role in entrainment under more naturalistic lighting conditions (eg, regimens including twilight transitions, seasonally changing photoperiod, or simulated moonlight), relative to the square-wave light-dark cycles commonly used in the laboratory.[72]

In addition to providing a secondary, indirect source of photic signaling to the circadian clock, the IGL also plays a preeminent role in the regulation of the circadian system by nonphotic, arousal-related stimuli. Thus, IGL lesions abolish the phase-shifting effects of novelty induced wheel running and benzodiazepine administration in hamsters, as well as the period-shortening effect of running-wheel access in rats and the entrainment effect of scheduled daily treadmill activity in mice.[73–78] More recently, evidence has been presented that IGL neurons may mediate the effects of metabolic signals on the SCN pacemaker.[79,80]

A third major afferent system converging mainly on the SCN core originates from the serotonergic midbrain raphe, especially the median raphe nucleus[81–84] (see **Fig. 1**). In addition, ascending serotonergic projections originating in the dorsal raphe nucleus innervate the IGL, providing a second route for serotonergic regulation of the SCN circadian pacemaker.[81,82] As for the IGL itself, extensive evidence has implicated serotonergic projections to the SCN and IGL in modulation of photic effects on the circadian pacemaker, as well as in the mediation of nonphotic effects on the pacemaker. These effects seem to be mediated via 5-hydroxytryptamine (5-HT)$_{1A}$ and 5-HT$_7$

receptors within the SCN, the IGL, and the raphe nuclei, and by 5-HT$_{1B}$ receptors located presynaptically on RHT terminals.[85–89]

In addition to the RHT, GHT, and 5-HT projections, several other identified pathways provide afferent input to the circadian system, including noradrenergic projections from the locus coeruleus, cholinergic projections from the basal forebrain and pontine tegmentum, and histaminergic projections from the posterior hypothalamus.[90,91] Like serotonergic projections, noradrenergic and cholinergic projections also innervate the IGL, providing an alternate pathway by which these transmitter systems could alter SCN function. However, unlike the RHT, GHT, and 5-HT projections to the SCN, which form generally overlapping terminal fields in the SCN core, noradrenergic, cholinergic, and histaminergic SCN inputs preferentially target the SCN shell. Beyond these systems, a recent review concluded that the SCN receives direct monosynaptic projections from at least 35 distinct brain areas,[41] revealing enormous potential for circadian pacemaker modulation by a wide range of extrinsic and intrinsic stimuli.

SUPRACHIASMATIC NUCLEUS OUTPUT PATHWAYS

Perhaps surprisingly, first-order SCN efferents innervate a relatively small number of target areas concentrated mainly in the diencephalon and basal forebrain.[92,93] These SCN targets then relay circadian timing signals to autonomic and neuroendocrine systems, as well as to central structures regulating affective, sensory, and motor processes, as well as to sleep-regulatory brain regions.[94] SCN efferents emerge from both the core and shell subnuclei and release several neurotransmitters and peptides including GABA, glutamate, and vasopressin (see **Fig. 1**). Remarkably, anatomically distinct populations of SCN neurons seem to innervate specific efferent targets, providing multiple waves of neuronal signals that regulate circadian phase in a target-specific manner. Despite earlier evidence that neuronal efferents were exclusively responsible for conveying SCN output signals,[95] it now appears that the SCN regulates certain rhythmic processes via diffusible paracrine signals. Evidence for a diffusible SCN output signal was first suggested by the finding that surgical isolation of the hamster SCN within a hypothalamic island abolished SCN-dependent neuroendocrine responses but allowed for persisting locomotor activity rhythms in the same animals.[96] The hypothesis for paracrine signaling from the SCN in the regulation of rhythmic processes was strengthened considerably by the finding that transplant of SCN tissue encased within a semipermeable capsule could restore locomotor but not neuroendocrine rhythms to SCN-lesioned arrhythmic hosts.[97] Several diffusible candidate molecules have now been implicated as circadian output signals, including prokineticin-2, tumor necrosis factor-α, and vasopressin.[97]

MULTIOSCILLATOR NATURE OF THE CIRCADIAN SYSTEM

The evidence reviewed above amply justifies the use of the term pacemaker to describe the SCN's role in circadian rhythmicity. Nevertheless, the larger circadian system is now known to be composed of a multiplicity of circadian oscillators distributed widely in the brain and body. Although extensive physiologic studies conducted in the premolecular era revealed several varieties of rhythmic dissociation and disruption that strongly implied the existence of a multioscillatory circadian system,[98] these studies provided little evidence regarding the anatomic localization and distribution of the circadian system.

After the elucidation of the core clock genes, it soon became apparent that the expression of these genes was not restricted to the SCN but was in fact widely distributed in the brain and periphery. Nevertheless, it was generally believed that non-SCN cellular oscillators were highly damped and possessed little or no capacity for self-sustainment in the absence of periodic SCN input. More recently, however, the finding that circadian clock genes express persistent rhythmically in several surgically isolated brain regions[99,100] and in numerous cultured peripheral tissues and cell types[101,102] has provided compelling evidence for a whole-body, anatomically distributed network of cellular- and tissue-level circadian clocks. Thus, the current conception of the circadian system is that the SCN pacemaker entrains rhythmicity in downstream central and peripheral clocks via neural and neuroendocrine signals, as well as less directly via its control of rhythmic feeding, activity, and body temperature,[103] which in turn entrain other behavioral, physiologic, and cellular rhythms (**Fig. 2**). In this way, a broad network of direct and indirect controls ensures that the SCN and other central and peripheral clocks maintain specific, and presumably optimal, phase relationships with the external and internal environment, resulting in the overall temporal coordination of the system.

What is the advantage of a distributed system of independent circadian clocks, as opposed to a passive system that strongly depends on SCN signals for the sustainment of periodicity? Perhaps

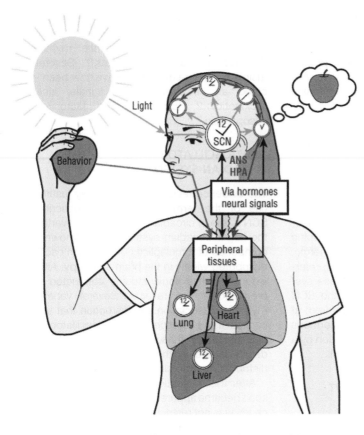

Fig. 2. The multioscillatory circadian timing system includes a large number of autonomously rhythmic circadian clock cells distributed within both central and peripheral tissues. The circadian pacemaker resides in the SCN, is entrained by light-dark cycles and other environmental stimuli, and in turn, serves to entrain and synchronize peripheral clocks. While some peripheral tissues can exhibit persistent autonomous rhythmicity, others may be damped in the absence of periodic SCN signals. Together, SCN and non-SCN central neural oscillators result in rhythmic behavior (such as food intake and motor activity), autonomic nervous system (ANS) function, and hypothalamic-pituitary-adrenal (HPA) axis hormone secretion. These behavioral and physiologic rhythms in turn can give rise to other rhythmic signals (eg, glucose availability, corticosterone levels, and body temperature) that serve to maintain phase synchrony among peripheral oscillators, probably in a tissue-specific manner. In turn, the activity of peripheral oscillators may give rise to rhythmic signals (eg, peripheral hormones, autonomic afferents, and metabolic signals) that contribute to the synchronization of the SCN pacemaker and other central oscillators.

the advantage lies in the ability of such a system to display a degree of plasticity in internal phase relationships under certain environmental conditions, such as when sleep and wakefulness occur at abnormal clock times or when feeding is restricted to atypical temporal windows. Under such conditions, a system of largely self-sustaining clocks can maintain largely undamped rhythmicity at the cellular and tissue levels. Thus, although temporal coordination throughout the circadian system is generally assumed to be physiologically optimal, the overall circadian system may be designed to allow downstream oscillators to display adaptive phase adjustments under certain natural circumstances. Of course, such plasticity may become maladaptive when humans choose to chronically disconnect their feeding and/or sleep-wake cycles from the SCN, as so often occurs in the current 24/7 society.

THE CIRCADIAN TIMING SYSTEM IN HEALTH AND DISEASE

This new picture of the circadian timing system has raised important questions about the potential

adverse health effects that may be associated with a loss of normal synchronization between and among central and peripheral oscillations. Thus, circadian disruption at the molecular and systemic levels has been linked to sleep disorders, obesity and diabetes, heart disease, cancer, and psychiatric disorders.[103–106] Given estimates that approximately 10% to 20% of the entire genome is expressed rhythmically in any given tissue or organ,[107,108] many other mechanisms linking circadian synchrony and desynchrony to health and disease will undoubtedly emerge in the next few years and beyond.

Circadian dysregulation certainly occurs quite often in humans, who can override their circadian clock and exert substantial volitional control over their sleep-wake and feeding cycles. Under such circumstances, abnormal phase relationships are expressed between sleep-wake behaviors (and other rhythmic processes tightly linked to sleep or wake states, as well as feeding or fasting states) and the circadian clock (and rhythmic processes tightly linked to those behavioral processes). Although the internal desynchronies that occur with jet lag and shift work may be the most dramatic, they are not the only examples of real-world circadian disruption. Indeed, social constraints, work schedules, and the use of artificial lighting may result in the widespread occurrence of social jet lag even in people living under relatively stable entrained conditions but who phase shift their sleep and feeding times on weekends and holidays relative to the weekdays.[109] Regardless of work or travel schedules, humans in the modern, round-the-clock society are certainly becoming less strictly diurnal, opposing millions of years of evolutionary selection.

SUMMARY

The SCN contains a master circadian pacemaker that entrains, coordinates, and contributes to the sustainment of a large population of cellular- and tissue-level circadian clocks located throughout the brain and body. Furthermore, the SCN itself contains a large number of normally coupled, but potentially autonomous, cellular oscillators that interact to underlie its pacemaker function. These cellular oscillations are generated by a set of circadian clock genes that interact via negative and positive feedback and ultimately drive circadian expression of a large number of clock-controlled genes, which in turn regulate downstream cellular and physiologic processes. Anatomically, the SCN is characterized by a complex regional organization that is not fully understood. The SCN pacemaker is entrained by several convergent afferent pathways that signal photic and nonphotic stimuli that mediate pacemaker entrainment to periodic environmental events. SCN outputs serve to synchronize non-SCN clocks and to impose rhythmicity on otherwise nonrhythmic processes. While it is becoming increasingly clear that proper coordination of the overall circadian system is critical for maintenance of health and well-being, it may also be the case that adaptive uncoupling among circadian clocks may allow for temporal adaptation to challenging environments.

REFERENCES

1. Moore RY, Eichler VB. Loss of a circadian adrenal corticosterone rhythm following suprachiasmatic lesions in the rat. Brain Res 1972;42(1):201–6.
2. Stephan FK, Zucker I. Circadian rhythms in drinking behavior and locomotor activity of rats are eliminated by hypothalamic lesions. Proc Natl Acad Sci U S A 1972;69(6):1583–6.
3. Weaver DR. The suprachiasmatic nucleus: a 25-year retrospective. J Biol Rhythms 1998;13(2):100–12.
4. Welsh DK, Logothetis DE, Meister M, et al. Individual neurons dissociated from rat suprachiasmatic nucleus express independently phased circadian firing rhythms. Neuron 1995;14:697–706.
5. Herzog ED, Geusz ME, Khalsa SB, et al. Circadian rhythms in mouse suprachiasmatic nucleus explants on multimicroelectrode plates. Brain Res 1997;757:285–90.
6. Colwell CS. Circadian modulation of calcium levels in cells in the suprachiasmatic nucleus. Eur J Neurosci 2000;12:571–6.
7. Kuhlman SJ, Quintero JE, McMahon DG. GFP fluorescence reports Period 1 gene regulation in the mammalian biological clock. Neuroreport 2000;11:1479–82.
8. Low-Zeddies SS, Takahashi JS. Chimera analysis of the Clock mutation in mice shows that complex cellular integration determines circadian behavior. Cell 2001;105:25–42.
9. Shirakawa T, Honma S, Honma K. Multiple oscillators in the suprachiasmatic nucleus. Chronobiol Int 2001;18:371–87.
10. Yamaguchi S, Isejima H, Matsuo T, et al. Synchronization of cellular clocks in the suprachiasmatic nucleus. Science 2003;302:1408–12.
11. Welsh DK, Takahashi JS, Kay SA. Suprachiasmatic nucleus: cell autonomy and network properties. Annu Rev Physiol 2010;72:551–77.
12. Mohawk JA, Takahashi JS. Cell autonomy and synchrony of suprachiasmatic nucleus circadian oscillators. Trends Neurosci 2011;34:349–58.
13. Schwartz W, Gross RA, Morton MT. The suprachiasmatic nuclei contain a tetrodotoxin-resistant circadian pacemaker. Proc Natl Acad Sci U S A 1987;84:1694–8.
14. Shibata S, Moore RY. Tetrodotoxin does not affect circadian rhythms in neuronal activity and metabolism in rodent suprachiasmatic nucleus in vitro. Brain Res 1993;606:259–66.
15. Miche S, Colwell CS. Cellular communication and coupling within the suprachiasmatic nucleus. Chronobiol Int 2001;18:579–600.
16. Aton SJ, Herzog ED. Come together, right … now: synchronization of rhythms in a mammalian circadian clock. Neuron 2005;48:531–4.
17. Herzog ED. Neurons and networks in daily rhythms. Nat Rev Neurosci 2007;8:790–802.
18. Takahashi JS, Turek FW. Anisomycin, an inhibitor of protein synthesis, perturbs the phase of a mammalian circadian pacemaker. Brain Res 1987;405:199–203.
19. Inouye ST, Takahashi JS, Wollnik F, et al. Inhibitor of protein synthesis phase shifts a circadian pacemaker in the mammalian SCN. Am J Physiol 1988;255:R1055–8.
20. Vitaterna MH, King DP, Chang A-M, et al. Mutagenesis and mapping of a mouse gene, Clock,

essential for circadian behavior. Science 1994;264:719–25.

21. Allada R, Emery P, Takahashi JS, et al. Stopping time: the genetics of fly and mouse circadian clocks. Annu Rev Neurosci 2001;24:1091–119.

22. Ko CH, Takahashi JS. Molecular components of the mammalian circadian clock. Hum Mol Genet 2006;15:R271–7.

23. Debruyne JP, Noton E, Lambert CM, et al. A clock shock: mouse CLOCK is not required for circadian oscillator function. Neuron 2006;50:465–77.

24. DeBruyne JP, Weaver DR, Reppert SM. CLOCK and NPAS2 have overlapping roles in the suprachiasmatic circadian clock. Nat Neurosci 2007;10:543–5.

25. Shearman LP, Zylka MJ, Weaver DR, et al. Two period homologs: circadian expression and photic regulation in the suprachiasmatic nuclei. Neuron 1997;19:1261–9.

26. Zheng B, Albrecht U, Kaasik K, et al. Nonredundant roles of the mPer1 and mPer2 genes in the mammalian circadian clock. Cell 2001;105:683–94.

27. Miyamoto Y, Sancar A. Circadian regulation of cryptochrome genes in the mouse. Brain Res Mol Brain Res 1999;71:238–43.

28. Van der Horst GT, Muijtjens M, Kobayashi K, et al. Mammalian Cry1 and Cry2 are essential for maintenance of circadian rhythms. Nature 1999;398:627–30.

29. Lowrey PL, Shimomura K, Antoch MP, et al. Positional syntenic cloning and functional characterization of the mammalian circadian mutation tau. Science 2000;288:483–92.

30. Meng QJ, Logunova L, Maywood ES, et al. Setting clock speed in mammals: the CK1 epsilon tau mutation in mice accelerates circadian pacemakers by selectively destabilizing PERIOD proteins. Neuron 2008;58:78–88.

31. Godinho SI, Maywood ES, Shaw L, et al. The after-hours mutant reveals a role for Fbxl3 in determining mammalian circadian period. Science 2007;316:897–900.

32. Siepka SM, Yoo SH, Park J, et al. Circadian mutant Overtime reveals F-box protein FBXL3 regulation of cryptochrome and period gene expression. Cell 2007;129:1011–23.

33. Maywood ES, Chesham JE, Meng QJ, et al. Tuning the period of the mammalian circadian clock: additive and independent effects of CK1epsilonTau and Fbxl3Afh mutations on mouse circadian behavior and molecular pacemaking. J Neurosci 2010;31:1539–44.

34. Colwell CS. Linking neural activity and molecular oscillations in the SCN. Nat Rev Neurosci 2010;12:553–69.

35. Naylor E, Bergmann BM, Krauski K, et al. The circadian clock mutation alters sleep homeostasis in the mouse. J Neurosci 2000;20:8138–43.

36. Tafti M, Franken P. Functional genomics of sleep and circadian rhythm. Invited review: genetic dissection of sleep. J Appl Physiol 2002;92:1339–47.

37. Rosenwasser AM. Circadian clock genes: non-circadian roles in sleep, addiction, and psychiatric disorders? Neurosci Biobehav Rev 2010;34:1249–55.

38. Moore RY. Entrainment pathways and the functional organization of the circadian system. Prog Brain Res 1996;111:103–19.

39. Moore RY, Silver R. Suprachiasmatic nucleus organization. Chronobiol Int 1998;15:475–87.

40. Morin LP. SCN organization reconsidered. J Biol Rhythms 2007;22:3–13.

41. Morin LP. Neuroanatomy of the extended circadian rhythm system. Exp Neurol 2013;243:4–20.

42. Antle MC, Silver R. Orchestrating time: arrangements of the brain circadian clock. Trends Neurosci 2005;28:145–51.

43. Shinohara K, Honma S, Katsuno Y, et al. Two distinct oscillators in the rat suprachiasmatic nucleus in vitro. Proc Natl Acad Sci U S A 1995;92:7396–400.

44. de la Iglesia HO, Cambras T, Schwartz WJ, et al. Forced desynchronization of dual circadian oscillators within the rat suprachiasmatic nucleus. Curr Biol 2004;14:796–800.

45. Johnson RF, Moore RY, Morin LP. Loss of entrainment and anatomical plasticity after lesions of the hamster retinohypothalamic tract. Brain Res 1998;460:297–313.

46. Golombek DA, Rosenstein RE. Physiology of circadian entrainment. Physiol Rev 2010;90:1063–102.

47. Moore RY, Speh JC, Card JP. The retinohypothalamic tract originates from a distinct subset of retinal ganglion cells. J Comp Neurol 1995;352:351–66.

48. Johnson RF, Morin LP, Moore RY. Retinohypothalamic projects in the hamster and rat demonstrated using cholera toxin. Brain Res 1998;462:301–12.

49. Levine JD, Weiss ML, Rosenwasser AM, et al. Retinohypothalamic tract in the female albino rat: a study using horseradish peroxidase conjugated to cholera toxin. J Comp Neurol 1991;306:344–60.

50. Foster RG, Argamaso S, Coleman S, et al. Photoreceptors regulating circadian behavior: a mouse model. J Biol Rhythms 1993;8(Suppl):S17–23.

51. Freedman MS, Lucas RJ, Soni B, et al. Regulation of mammalian circadian behavior by non-rod, non-cone, ocular photoreceptors. Science 1999;284:502–4.

52. Hattar S, Liao HW, Takao M, et al. Melanopsin-containing retinal ganglion cells: architecture, projections, and intrinsic photosensitivity. Science 2002;295:1065–70.

53. Berson DM, Dunn FA, Takao M. Phototransduction by retinal ganglion cells that set the circadian clock. Science 2002;295:1070–3.

54. Ruby NF, Brennan TJ, Xie X, et al. Role of melanopsin in circadian responses to light. Science 2002; 298:2211–3.

55. Panda S, Sato TK, Castrucci AM, et al. Melanopsin (Opn4) requirement for normal light-induced circadian phase shifting. Science 2002;298:2213–6.

56. Hattar S, Lucas RJ, Mrosovsky N, et al. Melanopsin and rod-cone photoreceptive systems account for all major accessory visual functions in mice. Nature 2003;424:76–81.

57. Drouyer E, Rieux C, Hut RA, et al. Responses of suprachiasmatic nucleus neurons to light and dark adaptation: relative contributions of melanopsin and rod-cone inputs. J Neurosci 2007;27:9623–31.

58. Guler AD, Altimus CM, Ecker JL, et al. Multiple photoreceptors contribute to nonimage-forming visual functions predominantly through melanopsin-containing retinal ganglion cells. Cold Spring Harb Symp Quant Biol 2007;72:509–15.

59. Gillette MU. Regulation of entrainment pathways by the suprachiasmatic circadian clock: sensitivities to second messengers. Prog Brain Res 1996;111:121–32.

60. Kornhauser JM, Ginty DD, Greenberg ME, et al. Light entrainment and activation of signal transduction pathways in the SCN. Prog Brain Res 1996; 111:133–46.

61. Shigeyoshi Y, Taguchi K, Yamamoto S, et al. Light-induced resetting of a mammalian circadian clock is associated with rapid induction of the mPer1 transcript. Cell 1997;91:1043–53.

62. Moriya T, Horikawa K, Akiyama M, et al. Correlative association between N-methyl-D-aspartate receptor-mediated expression of period genes in the suprachiasmatic nucleus and phase shifts in behavior with photic entrainment of clock in hamsters. Mol Pharmacol 2000;58:1554–62.

63. Challet E, Dugovic C, Turek FW, et al. The selective neurokinin 1 receptor antagonist R116301 modulates photic responses of the hamster circadian system. Neuropharmacology 2001;40:408–15.

64. Kim DY, Kang HC, Shin HC, et al. Substance P plays a critical role in photic resetting of the circadian pacemaker in the rat hypothalamus. J Neurosci 2001;21: 4026–31.

65. Piggins HD, Rusak B. Effects of microinjections of substance P into the suprachiasmatic nucleus region on hamster wheel-running rhythms. Brain Res Bull 1997;42:451–5.

66. Chen D, Buchanan GF, Ding JM, et al. Pituitary adenylate cyclase-activating peptide: a pivotal modulator of glutamatergic regulation of the suprachiasmatic circadian clock. Proc Natl Acad Sci U S A 1999;96: 13468–73.

67. Harrington ME, Hoque S, Hall A, et al. Pituitary adenylate cyclase activating peptide phase shifts circadian rhythms in a manner similar to light. J Neurosci 1999;19:6637–42.

68. Hannibal J, Jamen F, Nielsen HS, et al. Dissociation between light-induced phase shift of the circadian rhythm and clock gene expression in mice lacking the pituitary adenylate cyclase activating polypeptide type 1 receptor. J Neurosci 2001;21:4883–90.

69. Moore RY, Card JP. Intergeniculate leaflet: an anatomically and functionally distinct subdivision of the lateral geniculate complex. J Comp Neurol 1994;344:403–30.

70. Morin LP. The circadian visual system. Brain Res Rev 1994;67:102–27.

71. Harrington ME. The ventral lateral geniculate nucleus and the intergeniculate leaflet: interrelated structures in the visual and circadian systems. Neurosci Biobehav Rev 1997;21:705–27.

72. Pickard GE. Bifurcating axons of retinal ganglion cells terminate in the hypothalamic suprachiasmatic nucleus and in the intergeniculate leaflet of the thalamus. Neurosci Lett 1982;55:211–7.

73. Wickland CR, Turek FW. Lesions of the thalamic intergeniculate leaflet block activity-induced phase shifts in the circadian activity rhythm of the golden hamster. Brain Res 1994;660:293–300.

74. Janik D, Mrosovsky N. Intergeniculate leaflet lesions and behaviorally-induced shifts of circadian rhythms. Brain Res 1994;651:174–82.

75. Johnson R, Smale L, Moore RY, et al. Lateral geniculate lesions block circadian phase-shift responses to a benzodiazepine. Proc Natl Acad Sci U S A 1988;85:5301–4.

76. Meyer EL, Harrington ME, Rahmani T. A phase-response curve to the benzodiazepine chlordiazepoxide and the effect of geniculo-hypothalamic tract ablation. Physiol Behav 1993;53:237–43.

77. Kuroda H, Fukushima M, Nakai M, et al. Daily wheel running activity modifies the period of free-running rhythm in rats via intergeniculate leaflet. Physiol Behav 1997;61:633–7.

78. Marchant EG, Watson NV, Mistlberger RE. Both neuropeptide Y and serotonin are necessary for entrainment of circadian rhythms in mice by daily treadmill running schedules. J Neurosci 1997;17: 7974–87.

79. Pekala D, Blasiak T, Raastad M, et al. The influence of orexins on the firing rate and pattern of rat intergeniculate leaflet neurons–electrophysiological and immunohistological studies. Eur J Neurosci 2011;34:1406–18.

80. Saderi N, Cazarez-Marquez F, Buijs FN, et al. The NPY intergeniculate leaflet projections to the suprachiasmatic nucleus transmit metabolic conditions. Neuroscience 2013;246:291–300.

81. Meyer-Bernstein EL, Morin LP. Differential serotonergic innervation of the suprachiasmatic nucleus and the intergeniculate leaflet and its role in circadian rhythm modulation. J Neurosci 1996;16: 2097–111.

82. Morin LP. Serotonin and the regulation of mammalian circadian rhythmicity. Ann Med 1999;31:12–33.

83. Rea MA, Pickard GE. Serotonergic modulation of photic entrainment in the Syrian hamster. Biol Rhythm Res 2000;31:284–314.

84. Mistlberger RE, Antle MC, Glass JD, et al. Behavioral and serotonergic regulation of circadian rhythms. Biol Rhythm Res 2000;31:240–83.

85. Ehlen JC, Grossman GH, Glass JD. In vivo resetting of the hamster circadian clock by 5-HT7 receptors in the suprachiasmatic nucleus. J Neurosci 2001;21:5351–7.

86. Mintz EM, Gillespie CF, Marvel CL, et al. Serotonergic regulation of circadian rhythms in Syrian hamsters. Neuroscience 1997;79:563–9.

87. Prosser RA. Serotonergic actions and interactions on the SCN circadian pacemaker: in vitro investigations. Biol Rhythm Res 2000;31:315–39.

88. Pickard GE, Rea MA. TFMPP, a 5HT1B receptor agonist, inhibits light-induced phase shifts of the circadian activity rhythm and c-Fos expression in the mouse suprachiasmatic nucleus. Neurosci Lett 1997;231:95–8.

89. Smith BN, Sollars PJ, Dudek FE, et al. Serotonergic modulation of retinal input to the mouse suprachiasmatic nucleus mediated by 5-HT1B and 5-HT7 receptors. J Biol Rhythms 2001;16:25–38.

90. Rosenwasser AM. Neurobiology of the mammalian circadian system: oscillators, pacemakers, and pathways. Prog Psychobiol Physiol Psychol 2003; 18:1–38.

91. Rosenwasser AM, Turek FW. Physiology of the mammalian circadian system. In: Kryger MH, Roth T, Dement WC, editors. Principles and practice of sleep medicine. 5th edition. St Louis (MO): Elsevier-Saunders; 2011. p. 390–401.

92. Kalsbeek A, Perreau-Lenz S, Buijs RM. A network of (autonomic) clock outputs. Chronobiol Int 2006; 23:521–35.

93. Kalsbeek A, Palm IF, La Fleur SE, et al. SCN outputs and the hypothalamic balance of life. J Biol Rhythms 2006;21:458–69.

94. Rosenwasser AM. Functional neuroanatomy of sleep and circadian rhythms. Brain Res Rev 2009;61:281–306.

95. LeSauter J, Silver R. Output signals of the SCN. Chronobiol Int 1998;15:535–50.

96. Hakim H, DeBernardo AP, Silver R. Circadian locomotor rhythms, but not photoperiodic responses, survive surgical isolation of the SCN in hamsters. J Biol Rhythms 1991;6:97–113.

97. Silver R, LeSauter J, Tresco PA, et al. A diffusible coupling signal from the transplanted suprachiasmatic nucleus controlling circadian locomotor rhythms. Nature 1996;382:810–3.

98. Rosenwasser AM, Adler NT. Structure and function in circadian timing systems: evidence for multiple coupled circadian oscillators. Neurosci Biobehav Rev 1986;10:431–48.

99. Abe M, Herzog ED, Yamazaki S, et al. Circadian rhythms in isolated brain regions. J Neurosci 2002;22:350–6.

100. Granados-Fuentes D, Tseng A, Herzog ED. A circadian clock in the olfactory bulb controls olfactory responsivity. J Neurosci 2006;26:12219–25.

101. Yoo SH, Yamazaki S, Lowrey PL, et al. PERIOD2::-LUCIFERASE real-time reporting of circadian dynamics reveals persistent circadian oscillations in mouse peripheral tissues. Proc Natl Acad Sci U S A 2004;101:5339–46.

102. Welsh DK, Yoo SH, Liu AC, et al. Bioluminescence imaging of individual fibroblasts reveals persistent, independently phased circadian rhythms of clock gene expression. Curr Biol 2004;14:2289–95.

103. Hastings MH, Reddy AB, Maywood ES. A clockwork web: circadian timing in brain and periphery, in health and disease. Nat Rev Neurosci 2003;4:649–61.

104. Takahashi JS, Hong HK, Ko CH, et al. The genetics of mammalian circadian order and disorder: implications for physiology and disease. Nat Rev Genet 2008;9:764–75.

105. Karatsoreos IN. Effects of circadian disruption on mental and physical health. Curr Neurol Neurosci Rep 2012;12:218–25.

106. Zelinski EL, Deibel SH, McDonald RJ. The trouble with circadian clock dysfunction: multiple deleterious effects on the brain and body. Neurosci Biobehav Rev 2014;40:80–101.

107. Akhtar RA, Reddy AB, Maywood ES, et al. Circadian cycling of the mouse liver transcriptome, as revealed by cDNA microarray, is driven by the suprachiasmatic nucleus. Curr Biol 2002;12:540–50.

108. Panda S, Antoch MP, Miller BH, et al. Coordinated transcription of key pathways in the mouse by the circadian clock. Cell 2002;109:307–20.

109. Wittmann M, Dinich J, Merrow M, et al. Social jetlag: misalignment of social and biological time. Chronobiol Int 2006;23:497–509.

Genetics of Circadian Rhythms

Tomas S. Andreani, BA, Taichi Q. Itoh, PhD, Evrim Yildirim, PhD, Dae-Sung Hwangbo, PhD, Ravi Allada, MD*

KEYWORDS

• Circadian • Genetics • Entrainment • Clock

KEY POINTS

- Circadian rhythms at the organismal level are driven by rhythmic expression of genes at the molecular level.
- The conserved architecture of these circadian clocks is based on a transcriptional feedback loop with posttranscriptional and posttranslational regulation.
- Tissue-specific clocks are synchronized to local time by environmental cues, such as light and food.
- Dysregulation of circadian rhythms through mutation or misalignment with environmental time is shown to contribute to a wide range of disease states.

INTRODUCTION

Almost all organisms organize their physiology, behavior, and metabolism according to the 24-hour solar cycle. Time-dependent changes in these parameters have evolved to allow plants and animals to maximize their fitness according to external cues. Internal "clocks" evoke a set of anticipatory responses to changes in their environment, which are referred to as circadian rhythms.

Circadian rhythms have four unique properties. First, these rhythms closely mirror the 24-hour solar day, hence the word "circadian," which comes from the Latin words "circa" (close or about) and "dian" (day). The second principle dictates that even if there are no exogenous cues present, periodic patterns are still shown[1] indicating that these rhythms result from an internal time-keeping system. Third, although circadian activity rhythms are derived from an endogenous clock, they can adjust to exogenous signals, such as light or heat. Finally, the periodicity of rhythms is stable across a wide range of temperatures, a property referred to as "temperature compensation."[2] For humans, the most prominent circadian rhythm is the 24-hour rhythm in the sleep-wake cycle.

Four widely divergent model systems have been historically used to study the genetics underlying circadian rhythms: (1) fruit flies (*Drosophila*), (2) fungi (*Neurospora*), (3) cyanobacteria, and (4) mouse.[3] The discoveries found using these models have facilitated the understanding of the mechanism behind circadian rhythms and their significance to biology and disease. Remarkably, animal clocks are well conserved from insects to mammals, revealing an important role in basic animal models to understand the mechanistic basis of human circadian rhythms.

THE MOLECULAR CLOCK

Phasic expression of genes drives the physiologic and behavioral manifestations of circadian rhythms at the organismal level. Nearly half of all protein-coding genes show circadian-dependent transcription in at least one tissue in mammals.[4] Although it is known that the specific genes that cycle are variable across species and tissue

Disclosure Statement: The authors have nothing to disclose.
Department of Neurobiology, Northwestern University, 2205 Tech Drive, Evanston, IL 60208, USA
* Corresponding author.
E-mail address: r-allada@northwestern.edu

Sleep Med Clin 10 (2015) 413–421
http://dx.doi.org/10.1016/j.jsmc.2015.08.007
1556-407X/15/$ – see front matter © 2015 Elsevier Inc. All rights reserved.

sleep.theclinics.com

dependent,[5,6] the mechanism that drives their phasic expression is consistent throughout the body and well conserved between species.[7,8]

Rhythmic expression of genes is accomplished through a cell intrinsic transcriptional/translational feedback loop (TTFL). The forward portion of the loop consists of transcription factors whose activity promotes the expression of genes that are the "negative" elements of the loop. Over the course of a day, levels of the negative arm increase until they are capable of translocating into the nucleus and repressing the activity of the positive arm. Once they are degraded, the positive arm is freed to restart the cycle. The activity of this loop creates a self-perpetuating oscillating pattern of gene expression with a near 24-hour period. Here we present the mechanistic details of the fruit fly clock because it is where the clock mechanism was first discovered, is highly conserved with the human clock, and led to the discovery of the first genes involved in human circadian rhythms.

The Drosophila Molecular Clock

In *Drosophila* the forward transcription loop consists of master transcription factors clock (dCLK) and cycle (dCYC), which heterodimerize and initiate transcription.[9,10] This is accomplished through binding to the E-boxes (CACGTG) at target promoters and activating them (**Fig. 1**).[7] The negative loop consists of period (PER)[11] and timeless (TIM),[12] which dimerize and accumulate slowly in the cytoplasm. In the morning, light causes TIM

degradation and without TIM, PER is less stable and both are degraded by a proteasome-dependent pathway.[13] During the evening, however, PER/TIM accumulate and translocate into nucleus.[7,14,15] Once in the nucleus PER-TIM dimer binds to CLK-CYC and inhibits their transcriptional activity (see **Fig. 1**).[15] This simple negative feedback loop serves as the core principle and primary feedback loop of a 24-hour biologic clock.

In addition to this canonical loop, there are secondary loops that interact with and modulate clock activity. Clockwork orange (CWO) binds directly to E boxes, preventing CLK/CYC enhanced gene expression.[7] PAR-domain protein 1ε (PDP1ε) and vrille (VRI) are two proteins that also act to regulate the forward loop.[16] These circadian proteins feedback to act on the *Clk* promoter with PDP1ε serving as an activator and VRI as an inhibitor (see **Fig. 1**). Lastly, the transcription factor Ecdysone-induced protein 75 has been found to repress *Clk* expression[17] and time-dependently enhance PER transcription.[18] These additional feedback loops support the function of the primary feedback loop.

The Mammalian Molecular Clock

Mammalian and *Drosophila* TTFLs are similar.[6] In mouse and human the forward loop consists of CLOCK (homolog of dCLK) and brain and muscle Arnt-like protein-1 (BMAL1, homolog of dCYC), which also form a heterodimeric transcriptional activator (see **Fig. 1**). PER and cryptochrome

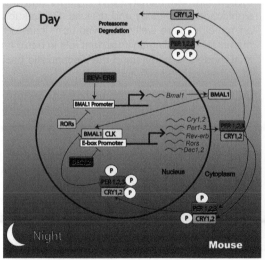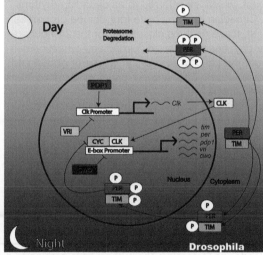

Fig. 1. Canonical molecular clocks in flies and mammals. Simplified *Drosophila* and mammalian circadian circuits. Arrows indicate activation and bars denote inhibition. Wavy lines represent rhythmic transcription. P marks phosphorylation. See text for more detail. BMAL1, brain and muscle Arnt-like protein-1; CRY, cryptochrome; CWO, clockwork orange; DEC, deleted in esophageal cancer; PDP, PAR-domain protein; PER, period; REV-ERB, reverse orientation c-erbA; ROR, retinoic acid related orphan receptor; TIM, timeless; VRI, vrille.

(CRY) homologs, of which there are three and two, respectively, are functionally homologous to PER and TIM in flies, respectively, and serve as the negative loop (see **Fig. 1**). *Drosophila* also uses a CRY that regulates transcription but also acts as a photosensor.

Although primary transcriptional and translational mechanisms for the molecular clocks are largely conserved, the paralogs add a layer of complexity. In *Drosophila* PER acts as the primary negative regulator. However, in mouse mPER1, mPER2, and mPER3 each play independent roles in the maintenance of molecular clocks.[19] An example of this is that mPER3 has a negligible role in circadian rhythms in the brain,[19] but plays a role in the regulation of circadian rhythms in peripheral tissues.[20] CRY paralogs show similar complexity with double knockout mutant mice for mCRY1 and mCRY2 displaying an arrhythmic phenotype, whereas a loss of function for one or the other results in either shortened or lengthened period by 1 hour, respectively.[21]

Secondary loops are also present in mammals, however, with added complexity. The mammalian equivalent to the *Drosophila* PDP1ε/VRI regulatory mechanism consists of receptors reverse orientation c-erbA (REV-ERB) and retinoic acid–related orphan receptor, which regulate the CLK heteromeric binding partner BMAL1, instead of CLK itself (see **Fig. 1**).[22] D-element binding protein and E4 binding protein 4 each bind to the promoter sequence (D-Box) of *mPer* and alter its expression pattern.[23] Finally, CLK-BMAL1 also facilitates expression of Deleted in esophageal cancer1,2 (*Dec1 Dec2*), the structural and functional homologs of CWO in flies. Similar to CWO, mammalian DEC1 and DEC2 also repress E-box targets including mPER and their own site thus forming an interlocked feedback loop (see **Fig. 1**).[24]

Posttranslational Modifications

Components of the TTFL are posttranslationally modified in a rhythmic manner to time their activity, subcellular localization, and/or stability. The major conserved mechanism of posttranslational modification is phosphorylation of the clock proteins (**Table 1**).[13]

In flies and mammals a key protein kinase is doubletime (DBT)/casein kinase (CK) 1 delta and epsilon (CK1δ/ε). In *Drosophila*, DBT binds to and phosphorylates PER, regulating its subcellular localization and signaling its rapid degradation by the proteasome.[25,26] The mammalian orthologs of DBT are CK1δ/ε, which mediate phosphorylation and degradation of mPER2 and facilitate its entry into the nucleus.[27] Thus, the CKI/PER

Table 1
Posttranslational modification

Posttranslational Modification	Target	Known Effects
Kinases		
CK1	PER1-2, CRY	Nuclear retention or degradation
DBT	dPER	Degradation and nuclear localization
CK2	dPER, PER2	Degradation and nuclear localization
Phosphatases		
PP1 (mammalian)	PER2	Nuclear localization and stabilization
PP1 (*Drosophila*)	dPER, TIM	Stabilization
PP2A	dPER	Nuclear localization

Abbreviations: CK, casein kinase; DBT, doubletime; PP, protein phosphatase.

relationship is conserved from flies to mammals. Even more remarkable is that mutations in CK1δ in humans cause familial advanced sleep phase disorder (FASPD).[28] Another critical kinase for PER activity is CK2, whose kinase activity promotes PER nuclear localization in mammalian and *Drosophila* cells.[29,30]

Phosphatases have been shown to modulate the clock. Protein phosphatase (PP) 1 dephosphorylates TIM, stabilizing it in the cytoplasm.[31] PP1 also acts on the phosphorylation state of PER itself.[32] In mammals, however, PP1 dephosphorylates PER2 stabilizing it for reentry into the nucleus.[33] The other major phosphatase involved in circadian rhythm modulation is PP2A.[34] Although the primary function of PP1 is stabilizing TIM and the PER/TIM complex, PP2A activity in *Drosophila* is involved in facilitating nuclear transport of PER/TIM through direct dephosphorylation of PER.[34]

MOLECULAR CLOCKS DRIVE PHYSIOLOGIC OUTPUT IN MULTICELLULAR ORGANISMS
Neural Circadian Networks

In multicellular organisms the circadian activity of master pacemakers in the brain govern the daily rhythms of sleep and wake. The discovery of the molecular clock and relevant circuitry has allowed for the exploration of this phenomenon in mammals and *Drosophila*.[6–8,35] In mammals a hypothalamic structure known as the suprachiasmatic nucleus (SCN) acts as the master timekeeper. The SCN is thought to entrain various parts of the body through its output to certain regions of the hypothalamus, which then signals the rest of the body and brain.[35,36] Drosophila behavioral rhythms are generated by the activity of approximately 150 interconnected pacemaker neurons in each brain hemisphere.[37] Independent groups within this network communicate with one another to integrate external cues and determine phase and period. Even in the highly divergent brains of insects and mammals, these clock neural networks consist of coupled oscillators.[37,38]

These master pacemakers drive behavioral rhythmicity via the rhythms of neuronal activity. Neuronal activity within the nuclei, in turn, is driven in part by the clock control of neuronal resting membrane potential. The resting membrane potential of clock neurons in Drosophila and mouse increases and decreases in a diurnal manner.[39,40] More positive resting membrane potential increases excitability and firing rates, whereas more negative potentials have the opposite effect.

Peripheral Tissues

In addition to the master circadian pacemakers in the brain, clocks are found in virtually every tissue and organ in flies and mammals. Clock genes are shown to be cycling in most nucleated mammalian cells except for the thymus and testis providing cyclic gene expression throughout the body.[35,41]

Some of the best-studied clocks in peripheral tissues are those in the pancreas and the liver because of their association with glucose homeostasis and metabolism. Mice with a pancreas-specific genetic inactivation of the essential clock component BMAL1 knockout show elevated glucose levels and impaired glucose tolerance and insulin secretion, suggesting a link between peripheral clock dysfunction and diabetes.[42] Similar tissue-specific knockout experiments in the liver showed the abolishment of the most clock-controlled gene expression despite continued input from the master circadian clock in the SCN.[43] These experiments and others demonstrate the significance of independent timing systems within the periphery whose regulation is critical for tissue function.

ENTRAINMENT OF THE CLOCK

To synchronize the clock to the 24-hour environment, organisms use sensory cues referred to as zeitgebers (German for "time giver" or "synchronizer"). Light and food are two well-studied zeitgebers that feedback to clock components to regulate their activity.

Light Entrainment

It is well known that most mammals receive visual input via retinal rod and cone photoreceptors, which send output to the retinal ganglion cells (RGC) that project into the brain. What is less well known and surprising is that rods and cones are not necessary for circadian entrainment. Mutant mice lacking rods and cones are still capable of entrainment to light-dark cycles.[44] Although most RGCs are incapable of directly perceiving light, a subset of them express the photopigment melanopsin, which responds to light independently of rod/cone system.[45] These intrinsically photosensitive RGCs send primarily glutamatergic and pituitary adenylate cyclase activating peptide outputs to the SCN.[46] Of note, flies also use nonvisual photoreceptors.[47] However, in an apparent point of divergence from mammals, flies also use CRY as a photoreceptor to synchronize brain circadian pacemakers and peripheral tissue clocks.

Glutamate-mediated effects on the clock genes within the SCN are well understood. Blockage of the glutamate receptor N-methyl-D-aspartate (NMDA), using an NMDA antagonist block, has been shown to block light-induced phase shifts.[48] Glutamate-induced calcium influx through NMDA and voltage-gated calcium channels leads to activation of the transcription factor cAMP-response element binding protein (**Fig. 2**).[49] mPer1 and mPer2 contain cAMP response elements (CRE) in their promoters and alter their expression in response to photic stimulation.[50]

Food

Food quality/dietary composition and timing can directly entrain or influence molecular clocks specifically in peripheral tissues (**Box 1**). Time-restricted feeding, where feeding is restricted to a particular time of day, causes peripheral clocks, such as those in liver, to be entrained without altering SCN clocks.[51] High-fat diet (HFD) can also reprogram peripheral circadian clocks in mice.[52] Interestingly, this mechanism seems to affect behavioral rhythms without affecting core clock genes in brain.[53] HFD-mediated circadian reprogramming is facilitated by nutrient-dependent chromatin remodeling. HFD impairs chromatin recruitment of CLK-BMAL1 to their target genes while at the same time it recruits supplementary transcription factors, such as peroxisome proliferator-activated receptor γ and sterol regulatory element-binding protein 1, to their target gene promoters.[52] Peroxisome proliferator-activated receptor γ can directly repress transcription of CLK-BMAL1,[54] suppressing the endogenous clock

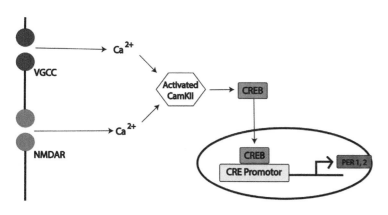

Fig. 2. Light input modulates clock gene expression in the SCN. Glutamatergic input to SCN activates NMDAR resulting in cascade to induce mPER1,2 expression. CamKII, Ca2+/calmodulin-dependent protein kinase II; CREB, Ca2+/cAMP response element-binding protein; NMDAR, N-methyl-D-aspartate receptor; VGCC; voltage-gated calcium channel.

while simultaneously transcribing a series of other non-clock-controlled genes.

The molecular clock is also directly influenced by nutrient-sensing/sensitive pathways. An example of this is the regulation of clock by nutrient responsive AMP-activated protein kinase (AMPK). Administration of AMPK activators, such as 5-aminoimidazole-4-carboxamide ribonucleotide (AICAR) and metformin, can reset the clock in mouse liver and activated AMPK mediates the degradation of CRY1.[55,56] Another example of this is the NAD^+-Sirtuin 1-CLOCK feedback loop. CLK-BMAL1 facilitates circadian expression of nicotinamide phosphoribosyltransferase, the rate-limiting enzyme for NAD^+ salvage pathways. NAD^+ also activates the deacetylase Sirtuin 1. This enzyme influences clock rhythms through interacting directly with PER2 and BMAL1, destabilizing PER2 and decreasing the activity of the negative arm of the TTFL.[36,57]

DYSREGULATION OF CLOCK AND DISEASE STATES

Endogenous molecular clocks can become out of phase with the environment or the rhythms of other tissues within the body. Clocks acting out of phase or desynchronized may exacerbate a wide range of disorders and diseases (**Fig. 3**).

Sleep

Circadian rhythms and sleep are inextricably linked. Sleep is a vital process linked to a myriad of processes including metabolism and synaptic plasticity.[58,59] PER mutations in mouse and human show that the circadian clock directly regulates the timing of sleep onset.[60] Mutation of various clock genes also inherently leads to abnormal sleep patterning and properties.[61,62] FASPD, a disorder in which individuals display approximately 4 hours earlier sleep and awaking times, is directly associated with *Per* mutations. Specifically PER phosphosite mutations[63,64] and mutations of CKI produce FASPD in humans.[28] Clock genes have also been implicated in regulating sleep duration. Mutations to DEC2 in humans and mice dice show increased wake and reduced rapid and non-rapid eye movement sleep states.[65]

Sleep timing and duration also have profound effects on the circadian clock. Insufficient sleep (sleep restriction) decreases the number of rhythmic genes in the human blood transcriptome compared with a control group with sufficient sleep.[66] Furthermore sleeping out of phase with the clock resulted in a six-fold reduction in the rhythmic transcripts in blood, not only because it results in lower amplitude of gene cycling, but also because there is suppression or enhancement of certain genes that manifest during sleep.[67] The application of genomic approaches could yield new diagnostic tests for circadian or sleep-based disorders.

Metabolism

Metabolic processes interact with central and peripheral clocks. One area where this has been explored extensively is in the context of metabolic diseases, specifically diabetes. *Clk* mutant mice tended to be hyperglycemic and have increased susceptibility to diet-induced obesity.[68] Pancreatic clock activity is directly involved in insulin release and β-cell health.[42] Work in other peripheral tissues, such as liver[69] and adipose tissue,[70] has furthered the idea that disruptions of CLK

Box 1
Nutrient intake modifies circadian rhythms

1. Food times provide entrainment mechanisms
2. Diet can modulate clock activity
3. Nutrient-sensitive pathways act directly on peripheral clocks to alter timing

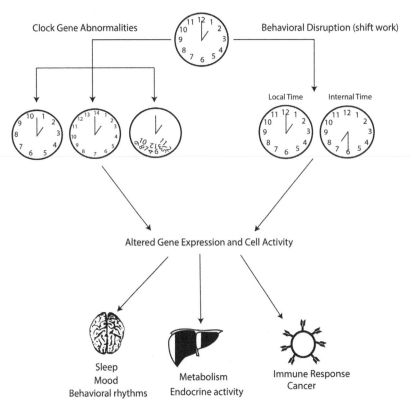

Fig. 3. Disruption of the molecular clock results in tissue-dependent disease states. Normal clock function aligns gene expression to a 24-hour cycle. Disruption of the genetic elements of tissue-specific clock results in diseases and disorders.

function may serve as a major culprit in metabolic syndrome.

In humans, CLK polymorphisms have been directly associated with obesity and metabolic syndrome.[71] Furthermore patients with type 2 diabetes showed down-regulation of *hPer2*, *hPer3*, and *hCry2* in their pancreatic islets relative to healthy patients.[72] Individuals who undergo shift work show increased rates of type 2 diabetes,[73] implicating disruption of circadian rhythms in the dramatic global increase of metabolic syndrome.

Cancer

Clock is involved in regulating a wide range of processes that are associated with cancer development including expression of numerous genes involved in DNA repair, cellular proliferation, and even tumorigenesis.[74] Furthermore, clock genes have been shown to be involved in the generation and progression of tumors. Ectopic expression of PER in human cancer cell lines results in growth inhibition, cell cycle arrest, and even apoptosis,[75] whereas targeted inhibition of PER has been shown to cause the induction of malignant lymphomas in mouse.[76]

Ovarian cancer cells show circadian-dependent S phase induction that is out of sync with that of the other human tissues.[77] *hPer1* shows lower expression levels in familial forms of breast cancer compared with sporadic forms[78] and dysregulation of the molecular clock has been directly associated with the progression of these cancers.[79] Disruption of the clock at the organismal level has been directly associated with increased risk of cancer in shift workers.[80] It is thought that disruption and dissociation of the peripheral and central clock mechanisms results in the unregulated cellular growth and activity characteristic to cancer (see **Fig. 3**).

Immune

Beyond the role in preventing disease states, clock may also be vital for combating them. Both quantity of immune cells and their gene expression are rhythmic.[81,82] Furthermore, mice display time-of-day-dependent responses to bacterial endotoxins and exotoxins, and proinflammatory cytokines.[83,84] Clock disruption studies have shown that T-cell antigen response is partially mediated by clock.[84]

Treatments

A wide range of treatments has emerged regarding circadian rhythms in humans. Pharmacologic methods center around melatonin, a rhythmically circulating hormone known to be important in the regulation of sleep and circadian rhythms. Melatonin directly affects the clock phase through activation of melatonin type 2 receptors[85] and is prescribed for numerous sleep disorders.[86] One of the more interesting directions circadian treatment is trending in is known as "chronotherapeutics." Treatments, such as those related to cancer, are applied with the timing dictated by the molecular clock, allowing therapeutic actions to be maximized according to the transcriptional state of the target.[87,88]

REFERENCES

1. Pittendrigh CS. Circadian rhythms and the circadian organization of living systems. Cold Spring Harb Symp Quant Biol 1960;25:159–84.
2. Eckardt NA. Temperature compensation of the circadian clock: a role for the morning loop. Plant Cell 2010;22(11):3506.
3. Rosbash M. The implications of multiple circadian clock origins. PLoS Biol 2009;7(3):e62.
4. Zhang R, Lahens NF, Ballance HI, et al. A circadian gene expression atlas in mammals: implications for biology and medicine. Proc Natl Acad Sci U S A 2014;111(45):16219–24.
5. Ko CH, Takahashi JS. Molecular components of the mammalian circadian clock. Hum Mol Genet 2006; 15(Spec No 2):R271–7.
6. Panda S, Hogenesch JB, Kay SA. Circadian rhythms from flies to human. Nature 2002;417(6886):329–35.
7. Allada R, Chung BY. Circadian organization of behavior and physiology in Drosophila. Annu Rev Physiol 2010;72:605–24.
8. Reppert SM, Weaver DR. Molecular analysis of mammalian circadian rhythms. Annu Rev Physiol 2001;63:647–76.
9. Allada R, White NE, So WV, et al. A mutant Drosophila homolog of mammalian clock disrupts circadian rhythms and transcription of period and timeless. Cell 1998;93(5):791–804.
10. Rutila JE, Suri V, Le M, et al. CYCLE is a second bHLH-PAS clock protein essential for circadian rhythmicity and transcription of Drosophila period and timeless. Cell 1998;93(5):805–14.
11. Konopka RJ, Benzer S. Clock mutants of Drosophila melanogaster. Proc Natl Acad Sci U S A 1971;68(9):2112–6.
12. Vosshall LB, Price JL, Sehgal A, et al. Block in nuclear localization of period protein by a second clock mutation, timeless. Science 1994;263(5153):1606–9.
13. Bae K, Edery I. Regulating a circadian clock's period, phase and amplitude by phosphorylation: insights from Drosophila. J Biochem 2006;140(5):609–17.
14. Curtin KD, Huang ZJ, Rosbash M. Temporally regulated nuclear entry of the Drosophila period protein contributes to the circadian clock. Neuron 1995;14(2):365–72.
15. Hardin PE. Molecular genetic analysis of circadian timekeeping in Drosophila. Adv Genet 2011;74:141–73.
16. Cyran SA, Buchsbaum AM, Reddy KL, et al. vrille, Pdp1, and dClock form a second feedback loop in the Drosophila circadian clock. Cell 2003;112(3):329–41.
17. Kumar S, Chen D, Jang C, et al. An ecdysone-responsive nuclear receptor regulates circadian rhythms in Drosophila. Nat Commun 2014;5:5697.
18. Jaumouille E, Machado Almeida P, Stahli P, et al. Transcriptional regulation via nuclear receptor crosstalk required for the Drosophila circadian clock. Curr Biol 2015;25(11):1502–8.
19. Bae K, Jin X, Maywood ES, et al. Differential functions of mPer1, mPer2, and mPer3 in the SCN circadian clock. Neuron 2001;30(2):525–36.
20. Pendergast JS, Oda GA, Niswender KD, et al. Period determination in the food-entrainable and methamphetamine-sensitive circadian oscillator(s). Proc Natl Acad Sci U S A 2012;109(35):14218–23.
21. van der Horst GT, Muijtjens M, Kobayashi K, et al. Mammalian Cry1 and Cry2 are essential for maintenance of circadian rhythms. Nature 1999;398(6728):627–30.
22. Lowrey PL, Takahashi JS. Mammalian circadian biology: elucidating genome-wide levels of temporal organization. Annu Rev Genomics Hum Genet 2004;5:407–41.
23. Cho C-H. Molecular mechanism of circadian rhythmicity of seizures in temporal lobe epilepsy. Front Cell Neurosci 2012;6:55.
24. Kato Y, Kawamoto T, Fujimoto K, et al. DEC1/STRA13/SHARP2 and DEC2/SHARP1 coordinate physiological processes, including circadian rhythms in response to environmental stimuli. Curr Top Dev Biol 2014;110:339–72.
25. Cyran SA, Yiannoulos G, Buchsbaum AM, et al. The double-time protein kinase regulates the subcellular localization of the Drosophila clock protein period. J Neurosci 2005;25(22):5430–7.
26. Price JL, Blau J, Rothenfluh A, et al. double-time is a novel Drosophila clock gene that regulates PERIOD protein accumulation. Cell 1998;94(1):83–95.
27. Akashi M, Tsuchiya Y, Yoshino T, et al. Control of intracellular dynamics of mammalian period proteins by casein kinase I epsilon (CKIepsilon) and

CKIdelta in cultured cells. Mol Cell Biol 2002;22(6): 1693–703.

28. Xu Y, Padiath QS, Shapiro RE, et al. Functional consequences of a CKIdelta mutation causing familial advanced sleep phase syndrome. Nature 2005; 434(7033):640–4.

29. Lin JM, Schroeder A, Allada R. In vivo circadian function of casein kinase 2 phosphorylation sites in Drosophila PERIOD. J Neurosci 2005;25(48): 11175–83.

30. Tsuchiya Y, Akashi M, Matsuda M, et al. Involvement of the protein kinase CK2 in the regulation of mammalian circadian rhythms. Sci Signal 2009; 2(73):ra26.

31. Fang Y, Sathyanarayanan S, Sehgal A. Post-translational regulation of the Drosophila circadian clock requires protein phosphatase 1 (PP1). Genes Dev 2007;21(12):1506–18.

32. Garbe DS, Fang Y, Zheng X, et al. Cooperative interaction between phosphorylation sites on PERIOD maintains circadian period in Drosophila. Plos Genet 2013;9(9):e1003749.

33. Schmutz I, Wendt S, Schnell A, et al. Protein phosphatase 1 (PP1) is a post-translational regulator of the mammalian circadian clock. PLoS One 2011; 6(6):e21325.

34. Sathyanarayanan S, Zheng X, Xiao R, et al. Post-translational regulation of Drosophila PERIOD protein by protein phosphatase 2A. Cell 2004;116(4): 603–15.

35. Hastings MH, Reddy AB, Garabette M, et al. Expression of clock gene products in the suprachiasmatic nucleus in relation to circadian behaviour. Novartis Found Symp 2003;253:203–17 [discussion: 102–9, 218–22, 281–4].

36. Froy O. Metabolism and circadian rhythms–implications for obesity. Endocr Rev 2010;31(1):1–24.

37. Nitabach MN, Taghert PH. Organization of the Drosophila circadian control circuit. Curr Biol 2008; 18(2):R84–93.

38. Pittendrigh CS, Daan S. Functional-analysis of circadian pacemakers in nocturnal rodents. 5. Pacemaker structure: clock for all seasons. J Comp Physiol 1976;106(3):333–55.

39. Colwell CS. Linking neural activity and molecular oscillations in the SCN. Nat Rev Neurosci 2011;12(10): 553–69.

40. Cao G, Nitabach MN. Circadian control of membrane excitability in Drosophila melanogaster lateral ventral clock neurons. J Neurosci 2008;28(25):6493–501.

41. Alvarez JD, Sehgal A. The thymus is similar to the testis in its pattern of circadian clock gene expression. J Biol Rhythms 2005;20(2):111–21.

42. Marcheva B, Ramsey KM, Buhr ED, et al. Disruption of the clock components CLOCK and BMAL1 leads to hypoinsulinaemia and diabetes. Nature 2010; 466(7306):627–31.

43. Kornmann B, Schaad O, Reinke H, et al. Regulation of circadian gene expression in liver by systemic signals and hepatocyte oscillators. Cold Spring Harb Symp Quant Biol 2007;72:319–30.

44. Freedman MS, Lucas RJ, Soni B, et al. Regulation of mammalian circadian behavior by non-rod, non-cone, ocular photoreceptors. Science 1999;284(5413): 502–4.

45. Berson DM, Dunn FA, Takao M. Phototransduction by retinal ganglion cells that set the circadian clock. Science 2002;295(5557):1070–3.

46. Hannibal J. Neurotransmitters of the retino-hypothalamic tract. Cell Tissue Res 2002;309(1): 73–88.

47. Veleri S, Rieger D, Helfrich-Forster C, et al. Hofbauer-Buchner eyelet affects circadian photosensitivity and coordinates TIM and PER expression in Drosophila clock neurons. J Biol rhythms 2007; 22(1):29–42.

48. Moriya T, Horikawa K, Akiyama M, et al. Correlative association between N-methyl-D-aspartate receptor-mediated expression of period genes in the suprachiasmatic nucleus and phase shifts in behavior with photic entrainment of clock in hamsters. Mol Pharmacol 2000;58(6):1554–62.

49. Tischkau SA, Mitchell JW, Tyan SH, et al. Ca2+/cAMP response element-binding protein (CREB)-dependent activation of Per1 is required for light-induced signaling in the suprachiasmatic nucleus circadian clock. J Biol Chem 2003;278(2):718–23.

50. Travnickova-Bendova Z, Cermakian N, Reppert SM, et al. Bimodal regulation of mPeriod promoters by CREB-dependent signaling and CLOCK/BMAL1 activity. Proc Natl Acad Sci U S A 2002;99(11): 7728–33.

51. Damiola F, Le Minh N, Preitner N, et al. Restricted feeding uncouples circadian oscillators in peripheral tissues from the central pacemaker in the suprachiasmatic nucleus. Genes Dev 2000;14(23):2950–61.

52. Eckel-Mahan K, Sassone-Corsi P. Metabolism and the circadian clock converge. Physiol Rev 2013; 93(1):107–35.

53. Kohsaka A, Laposky AD, Ramsey KM, et al. High-fat diet disrupts behavioral and molecular circadian rhythms in mice. Cell Metab 2007;6(5):414–21.

54. Fontaine C, Dubois G, Duguay Y, et al. The orphan nuclear receptor Rev-Erbalpha is a peroxisome proliferator-activated receptor (PPAR) gamma target gene and promotes PPARgamma-induced adipocyte differentiation. J Biol Chem 2003;278(39): 37672–80.

55. Lamia KA, Sachdeva UM, DiTacchio L, et al. AMPK regulates the circadian clock by cryptochrome phosphorylation and degradation. Science 2009; 326(5951):437–40.

56. Um JH, Pendergast JS, Springer DA, et al. AMPK regulates circadian rhythms in a tissue- and

isoform-specific manner. PLoS One 2011;6(3): e18450.

57. Asher G, Sassone-Corsi P. Time for food: the intimate interplay between nutrition, metabolism, and the circadian clock. Cell 2015;161(1):84–92.

58. Laposky AD, Bass J, Kohsaka A, et al. Sleep and circadian rhythms: key components in the regulation of energy metabolism. FEBS Lett 2008;582(1): 142–51.

59. Wright KP, Lowry CA, Lebourgeois MK. Circadian and wakefulness-sleep modulation of cognition in humans. Front Mol Neurosci 2012;5:50.

60. Jones CR, Huang AL, Ptacek LJ, et al. Genetic basis of human circadian rhythm disorders. Exp Neurol 2013;243:28–33.

61. Laposky A, Easton A, Dugovic C, et al. Deletion of the mammalian circadian clock gene BMAL1/Mop3 alters baseline sleep architecture and the response to sleep deprivation. Sleep 2005;28(4):395–409.

62. Naylor E, Bergmann BM, Krauski K, et al. The circadian clock mutation alters sleep homeostasis in the mouse. J Neurosci 2000;20(21):8138–43.

63. Toh KL, Jones CR, He Y, et al. An hPer2 phosphorylation site mutation in familial advanced sleep phase syndrome. Science 2001;291(5506):1040–3.

64. Xu Y, Toh KL, Jones CR, et al. Modeling of a human circadian mutation yields insights into clock regulation by PER2. Cell 2007;128(1):59–70.

65. He Y, Jones CR, Fujiki N, et al. The transcriptional repressor DEC2 regulates sleep length in mammals. Science 2009;325(5942):866–70.

66. Möller-Levet CS, Archer SN, Bucca G, et al. Effects of insufficient sleep on circadian rhythmicity and expression amplitude of the human blood transcriptome. Proc Natl Acad Sci 2013;110:E1132–41.

67. Archer SN, Laing EE, Möller-Levet CS, et al. Mistimed sleep disrupts circadian regulation of the human transcriptome. Proc Natl Acad Sci 2014; 111(6):E682–91.

68. Turek FW, Joshu C, Kohsaka A, et al. Obesity and metabolic syndrome in circadian Clock mutant mice. Science 2005;308(5724):1043–5.

69. Feng D, Liu T, Sun Z, et al. A circadian rhythm orchestrated by histone deacetylase 3 controls hepatic lipid metabolism. Science 2011;331(6022): 1315–9.

70. Paschos GK, Ibrahim S, Song WL, et al. Obesity in mice with adipocyte-specific deletion of clock component Arntl. Nat Med 2012;18(12):1768–77.

71. Scott EM, Carter AM, Grant PJ. Association between polymorphisms in the clock gene, obesity and the metabolic syndrome in man. Int J Obes (Lond) 2008;32(4):658–62.

72. Stamenkovic JA, Olsson AH, Nagorny CL, et al. Regulation of core clock genes in human islets. Metabolism 2012;61(7):978–85.

73. Gan Y, Yang C, Tong X, et al. Shift work and diabetes mellitus: a meta-analysis of observational studies. Occup Environ Med 2015;72(1):72–8.

74. Savvidis C, Koutsilieris M. Circadian rhythm disruption in cancer biology. Mol Med 2012;18:1249–60.

75. Gery S, Gombart AF, Yi WS, et al. Transcription profiling of C/EBP targets identifies Per2 as a gene implicated in myeloid leukemia. Blood 2005;106(8): 2827–36.

76. Fu L, Pelicano H, Liu J, et al. The circadian gene Period2 plays an important role in tumor suppression and DNA damage response in vivo. Cell 2002;111(1):41–50.

77. Klevecz RR, Shymko RM, Blumenfeld D, et al. Circadian gating of S phase in human ovarian cancer. Cancer Res 1987;47(23):6267–71.

78. Winter SL, Bosnoyan-Collins L, Pinnaduwage D, et al. Expression of the circadian clock genes Per1 and Per2 in sporadic and familial breast tumors. Neoplasia 2007;9(10):797–800.

79. Cadenas C, van de Sandt L, Edlund K, et al. Loss of circadian clock gene expression is associated with tumor progression in breast cancer. Cell Cycle 2014;13(20):3282–91.

80. Davis S, Mirick DK. Circadian disruption, shift work and the risk of cancer: a summary of the evidence and studies in Seattle. Cancer Causes Control 2006;17(4):539–45.

81. Born J, Lange T, Hansen K, et al. Effects of sleep and circadian rhythm on human circulating immune cells. J Immunol 1997;158(9):4454–64.

82. Mazzoccoli G, Sothern RB, Greco A, et al. Time-related dynamics of variation in core clock gene expression levels in tissues relevant to the immune system. Int J Immunopathol Pharmacol 2011;24(4): 869–79.

83. Scheiermann C, Kunisaki Y, Frenette PS. Circadian control of the immune system. Nat Rev Immunol 2013;13(3):190–8.

84. Fortier EE, Rooney J, Dardente H, et al. Circadian variation of the response of T cells to antigen. J Immunol 2011;187(12):6291–300.

85. Dubocovich ML, Rivera-Bermudez MA, Gerdin MJ, et al. Molecular pharmacology, regulation and function of mammalian melatonin receptors. Front Biosci 2003;8:d1093–108.

86. Pandi-Perumal SR, Trakht I, Spence DW, et al. The roles of melatonin and light in the pathophysiology and treatment of circadian rhythm sleep disorders. Nat Clin Pract Neurol 2008;4(8):436–47.

87. Levi F, Okyar A, Dulong S, et al. Circadian timing in cancer treatments. Annu Rev Pharmacol Toxicol 2010;50:377–421.

88. Scheer FA, Wright KP Jr, Kronauer RE, et al. Plasticity of the intrinsic period of the human circadian timing system. PLoS One 2007;2(8):e721.

Aging and Circadian Rhythms

Jeanne F. Duffy, MBA, PhD[a,b,*], Kirsi-Marja Zitting, PhD[a,b], Evan D. Chinoy, PhD[a,b]

KEYWORDS

- Aging • Circadian • Human • Light • Melatonin • Sleep

KEY POINTS

- Sleep timing changes with age.
- The circadian system is a major sleep regulatory system.
- There are age-associated changes in human circadian rhythms.
- There are age-associated changes in components of the circadian system in both animals and humans.
- There is evidence for alterations in circadian rhythmicity contributing to age-related changes in sleep.

INTRODUCTION

Earlier Sleep Timing and Reduced Sleep Consolidation with Age

A common feature of aging is the advance of the timing of sleep to earlier hours,[1–7] often earlier than desired.[8–10] The sleep of older people is also characterized by an increased number of awakenings[11] and a reduction of the deeper stages of non–rapid eye movement (REM) sleep (also called slow wave sleep [SWS], stages 3 and 4 sleep).[12–31] These age-related changes are also associated with sleep complaints, with most studies finding that more than one-third of older adults report early morning awakening and/or difficulty maintaining sleep on a regular (several times per week) basis.[8–10,32–34] Although sleep disorders are far more prevalent in older adults,[35] even otherwise healthy older individuals also show characteristic changes in sleep, including reductions in SWS and sleep efficiency and increases in awakenings.[36–40] Age-related changes in sleep structure are seen even in middle-aged adults.[36–40]

Circadian Timing System Regulates Sleep Timing and Consolidation

The circadian timing system is one of the 2 major sleep regulatory systems[41,42] (the other being a homeostatic sleep-wake process). The circadian timing system is a major determinant of the timing of sleep and sleep structure in humans, and many aspects of sleep vary markedly with circadian phase in both young and older adults.[43–46] A proper alignment between the timing of sleep and the circadian phase of sleep is important for sleep duration and quality, as demonstrated in both healthy subjects[47–49] and in some clinical conditions.[50,51] The circadian timing system has a major influence on the timing and duration of REM sleep[42] and has a smaller but still significant impact on many aspects of non-REM sleep. The

This work was supported in part by NIH grants P01 AG09975, R01 AG044416, and R01 HL094654. K.-M. Zitting is supported by a fellowship from the Finnish Cultural Foundation and a grant from the Gyllenberg Foundation; E.D. Chinoy is supported by a fellowship from institutional training grant T32 HL007901.
a Division of Sleep and Circadian Disorders, Departments of Medicine and Neurology, Brigham and Women's Hospital, 221 Longwood Avenue, BLI438, Boston, MA 02115, USA; b Division of Sleep Medicine, Harvard Medical School, Boston, MA, USA
* Corresponding author. Division of Sleep and Circadian Disorders, 221 Longwood Avenue, BLI438, Boston, MA 02115.
E-mail address: jduffy@hms.harvard.edu

Sleep Med Clin 10 (2015) 423–434
http://dx.doi.org/10.1016/j.jsmc.2015.08.002
1556-407X/15/$ – see front matter © 2015 Elsevier Inc. All rights reserved.

circadian drive for wakefulness increases across the biological day, reaching its maximum in the evening hours when homeostatic sleep pressure is high, the so-called wake-maintenance zone.[52,53] The circadian drive for sleep reaches its maximum during the early morning hours just before habitual awakening time, when homeostatic sleep pressure is low.[28,54] Under ideal conditions, the circadian rhythm of sleep-wake interacts with the homeostatic sleep-wake process to allow for consolidated sleep (and wake) in humans.[55–61] Studies in young adults have demonstrated that even a small change in the circadian time of sleep can have a large impact on the ability to consolidate sleep throughout the night. Thus, age-related changes in circadian rhythms or circadian sleep regulation may underlie the sleep timing and consolidation changes seen in aging and if so may be a target for therapeutics to improve sleep.

Circadian rhythms are endogenously generated oscillations in physiology and behavior with a near-24-hour period. Human circadian period averages slightly longer than 24 hours, with a range of about 23.5 to 24.5 hours in sighted adults.[62–68] The circadian system is synchronized to the 24-hour day by signals from the environment, a process called entrainment. In humans, as in most mammals, entrainment typically occurs via light-dark exposure. Light has a phase-dependent effect on the circadian system, meaning that the effect of a given light stimulus depends on the phase (or biological time of day) at which the light exposure occurs. Light exposure in the late evening and early night shifts the timing of rhythms later (phase delay shifts), light exposure in the late night and early morning shifts the timing of rhythms earlier (phase advance shifts), whereas light exposure in the middle of the biological day produces small changes in rhythm timing.[69,70] Plots of the magnitude of the phase shift with respect to the phase at which the light exposure was given are called phase response curves (PRCs). The phase relationship between the circadian system and the entraining signal is referred to as the phase angle (or phase angle of entrainment; **Fig. 1**). Circadian period interacts with the PRC in the entrainment process, and individuals with different periods (and/or different magnitude of PRCs) have different phase angles of entrainment.[68,71]

Age-related changes in any of the structures involved in generating or entraining circadian rhythms and/or age-related changes in any of the critical features or processes involved in entrainment may therefore contribute to altered circadian rhythm timing with advancing age. The evidence for alterations in circadian rhythms with age and

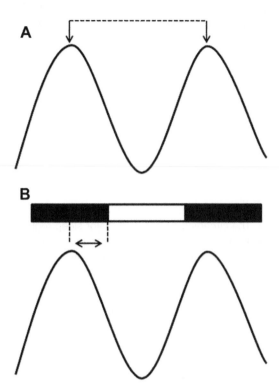

Fig. 1. Some key features of circadian rhythms. (*A*) Phase (*down arrows*) refers to a reference point in the approximately 24-hour rhythm, in this case the peak of the rhythm. The duration from the phase on one cycle to the same phase on the next cycle (*dashed line*) is the period (cycle length) of the rhythm. Period can be assessed only under controlled experimental conditions. (*B*) The near-24-hour circadian rhythms are entrained (synchronized) to the environment through periodic signals from the environment, typically light-dark exposure (*bar across the top of [B]*). The relationship between the entraining signal (here, lights on, *right dashed vertical line*) and the phase of the rhythm (here, the peak of the rhythm, *left dashed vertical line*) is referred to as the phase angle of entrainment (*horizontal arrow*). This phase angle depends on the period of the rhythm, the strength of the entraining signal, and the phase-dependent response to that entraining signal.

how these might contribute to age-related changes in sleep timing and consolidation are outlined in the following discussion.

Methods for Assessing Human Circadian Rhythms

Circadian phase is typically assessed in humans by measuring one or more of the physiologic parameters that are controlled in part by the circadian timing system. The most widely used measures of circadian phase in humans are the rhythms of core body temperature and melatonin (although many other hormones have rhythms), and each has its advantage and disadvantage. Body temperature has the advantage of being able to be collected continuously, whereas melatonin, which is typically measured in saliva or plasma, can be collected only at less frequent intervals (typically every 30–60 minutes). Body temperature can be measured using a rectal sensor or an ingestible transmitter. A major disadvantage of using body temperature as a marker of circadian timing is that the variations in temperature across the day are not only due to circadian rhythmicity but also due to factors such as posture, sleep-wake state, and activity level. Furthermore, the influence of those behavioral factors on body temperature is phase dependent, such that the change in temperature produced by the behavior is different depending on where in the circadian cycle the behavior occurs. Thus, diurnal variations in temperature, particularly the time of the nadir of the temperature cycle, may not reflect the underlying circadian variation. Melatonin has the advantage of being far less influenced by posture, sleep-wake state, and activity level than temperature, although there is some evidence that periodic changes in behavior can influence melatonin level. Melatonin is suppressed by light exposure, so ambient lighting must be strictly controlled at low levels throughout all sampling segments. One disadvantage of using melatonin as a circadian phase marker is that collection of samples during sleep may require interruption of sleep, although specialized blood collection systems used in many laboratories avoid sleep interruption. Because of this limitation, in many studies only the onset of melatonin secretion is used as a phase marker, rather than collection during the entire 24-hour rhythm. Although in many cases this dim-light melatonin onset is sufficient to determine changes in rhythm timing, it misses out on any changes in melatonin rhythm amplitude, duration, or offset timing.

The constant routine (CR) protocol was developed to assess the phase and amplitude of circadian rhythms.[72,73] The CR consists of a 24+ hour period of wakefulness in a semirecumbent posture, such that sleep-wake state, posture, and activity level are kept constant. Room temperature, humidity, and light level are similarly kept constant, and food and fluid intake are divided into small snacks that are consumed at regular intervals. In this way, many of the factors known to influence physiologic rhythms are either eliminated or are spread across day and night, allowing the underlying circadian oscillation to be observed. In studies of circadian rhythmicity in which sleep deprivation is a major concern, melatonin can be used as the sole circadian phase marker. Protocols in which 24 or more hours of data are collected under controlled conditions allow for assessment of circadian phase and amplitude, making the CR protocol ideal for such assessments.

Circadian period is typically assessed in animals by putting the animal into constant darkness and observing the rest-activity cycle over several days, whereas other methods are used to assess human circadian period. One method is the forced desynchrony (FD) protocol, in which the participant is scheduled to live on a rest-activity cycle much shorter or longer than 24 hours while continuous measurement of physiologic rhythms are collected.[62] FD data are then analyzed by accounting for the imposed periodicity resulting from the rest-activity cycle, while searching for periodicity within the circadian range. That method has been validated against period assessments from CRs and by multiple physiologic measures in the same individual showing the same periodicity.[62] Ultrashort sleep-wake cycles have been used to assess circadian period, although in most cases there has been no independent validation of this method of assessing period.

EVIDENCE FOR CIRCADIAN CHANGES IN AGING IN HUMANS
Circadian Phase

Circadian phase has been shown to move earlier, or advance, with age.[74–79] As described earlier, most rhythms controlled by the circadian system are also influenced by many external and behavioral factors, and therefore, the best evidence about circadian phase comes from studies conducted under laboratory conditions such as the CR, designed to control for effects of light exposure, posture, ambient temperature, sleep, and food intake.[73] The timing of the circadian rhythm of core body temperature has been reported to be earlier in both middle-aged and older (>60 years) adults than in young (20–30 years) adults.[1,76,80–83] The circadian phase of melatonin has also been reported to move earlier with age,[83–86] as has the timing of the cortisol rhythm.[78,79,87,88] **Fig. 2** illustrates the advanced phase observed in studies of older adults.

Phase of Entrainment

The phase relationship between a circadian rhythm of interest and the signal from the environment that entrains the rhythm (typically the light-dark cycle) is referred to as the phase angle of entrainment.[89] There is evidence from animals that the timing of the rhythm of locomotor activity

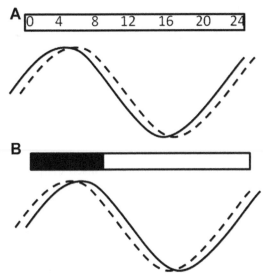

Fig. 2. Altered phase in older adults. (*A*) When compared with clock time (indicated in the bar across the *top of panel A*), the phase of both core body temperature and plasma melatonin is earlier in older adults (*solid line*) than it is in young adults (*dashed line*). (*B*) However, when compared with their usual sleep-wake and dark-light timing (sleep/dark indicated by the *horizontal black* bar, wake/light indicated by the *horizontal white* bar across the *top of panel B*), the phase of both core body temperature and plasma melatonin is later with respect to sleep/darkness in older adults (*solid line*) than it is in young adults (*dashed line*).

with respect to the timing of the light-dark cycle is altered in aging. Studies in hamsters found that activity onset is earlier with respect to lights out in older animals, and reentrainment after the light-dark cycle is shifted is faster.[90,91] However, a study in mice reported delayed activity onset and slower reentrainment.[92] Studies of phase angle in humans have either reported no difference with age[81,93–95] or found that older people show an altered phase angle, such that the timing of the phase of their rhythms of core body temperature and melatonin occur later with respect to sleep (and lights out).[1,84,85] This latter finding means that older adults are sleeping not only at an earlier clock time but also at an earlier biological time.

Circadian Amplitude

There are numerous reports of reduced circadian rhythm amplitude with aging. In animals, reduced amplitude of the rest-activity cycle[92,96–98] as well as the amplitude of multiunit electrical activity in the suprachiasmatic nucleus (SCN) have been reported.[99–102] In studies of human circadian rhythms, most reports find a reduced temperature

amplitude with age,[30,76,80,103] and many but not all find reduced amplitude of the rhythms of melatonin and other hormones.[6,94,104] Although changes in the electrical activity of the SCN likely lead to alterations in output rhythm amplitude, the functional consequences of alterations in output rhythm amplitude are not well understood.

Circadian-Sleep Interaction

As outlined earlier, the circadian system interacts with a sleep-wake homeostatic process to regulate the timing and consolidation of sleep in humans. Studies using protocols such as the FD protocol have been used to separate circadian from sleep-wake-dependent influences on sleep and waking performance and to compare those influences between young and older adults. Those studies have demonstrated that the sleep of older adults is much more vulnerable to circadian misalignment than the sleep of young adults.[11,28,30,31,37,46,105] There is a much narrower range of circadian times when the end of sleep can remain consolidated in older adults compared with young adults and a corresponding reduction in the range of circadian phases at which alertness and performance is impaired in older subjects,[1,60,106,107] suggesting an age-related reduction in the circadian drive for sleep in the early morning.[11,28,30,31,37,105] Studies using ultrashort sleep-wake cycles have also reported a reduction in the circadian drive for wakefulness in the evening (the wake-maintenance zone).[37,94] Together, these findings suggest that there may be a reduction in the circadian rhythm of sleep-wake propensity that occurs in aging.

Circadian Period

It was hypothesized that a shortening of circadian period with age could explain the shift in sleep timing with age, and there was evidence from some animal studies that the period was shorter in older animals.[108–110] An initial series of FD studies in which circadian period was assessed in healthy older adults and compared with young adults found no difference in period with age,[62] and in a follow-up study of a larger group of young and older adults the authors found the same result.[68] A study of 6 blind men who each had their period estimated twice during an approximately 10-year interval found no evidence for a shortening of period with age within an individual.[111] Together, these findings suggest that an age-related shortening of circadian period does not underlie the advance in circadian rhythms and sleep timing with age in humans.

Response to Light

Light is the primary environmental signal influencing circadian rhythms and serves to synchronize the near-24-hour circadian system to the 24-hour environmental day.[62–65,89,112–114] Most humans spend little time in outdoor levels of light,[115–117] and therefore, indoor light plays a dominant role in synchronizing circadian rhythms for most people. Use of artificial illumination in the evening has been shown to partially suppress and alter the timing of the melatonin rhythm and sleep in young adults.[118–121] Thus, the pattern of exposure to light in the evening is a likely mechanism contributing to circadian timing and sleep in older adults, and there is evidence to support age-related differences in light exposure patterns in older adults living in the community.[122,123]

Whether the response to light differs between young and older adults is also relevant to sleep and circadian rhythm timing, and several studies of the circadian response to light in older versus young adults have been carried out during the past 2 decades, with mixed findings. Klerman and colleagues[124] used a bright (10,000 lux) light stimulus of 5 hours/day over 3 days in young and older adults and delivered the light stimuli across the phase delay and the phase advance regions of the PRC. They found no evidence for an age difference in phase-shifting response when light was presented in the phase delay region and a suggestion that there might be reduced responses in the older participants in the phase advance region. Benloucif and colleagues[125] used a 4-hour 3500 lux stimulus delivered in the phase delay region and also found no evidence for an age difference in phase-shifting response. Kim and colleagues[83] tested a 2-hour light stimulus of 2000 or 8000 lux delivered at a variety of different phases and did not find significant differences in phase-shifting responses between young and older participants. Duffy and colleagues[126] used a 6.5-hour light stimulus in the phase delay region and tested a wide range of stimulus intensities. They found no difference in phase delay response for low (<100 lux) or high (>1000 lux) light levels but did find evidence for a reduced responsiveness among the older subjects in the intermediate range, with a half-maximal response shifted to 263 lux compared with 119 lux in the young adults.

Although all the previous studies used polychromatic light sources, additional studies using monochromatic light stimuli have also been conducted. Herljevic and colleagues[127] used a 30-minute light stimulus of short (456 nm) wavelength light delivered in the phase delay region and found significant differences in melatonin suppression between young and older women but no age difference when a longer (548 nm) wavelength light stimulus was used. In a study of 2 hours of intermittent short- or long-wavelength monochromatic light delivered in the phase advance region, Sletten and colleagues[128] reported that phase shifting responses were slightly larger in the young participants, although the difference was not statistically significant. Najjar and colleagues[129] studied a series of nonvisual responses to monochromatic light in young and older adults and found a shift in peak sensitivity to longer wavelengths in the older participants but no change in melatonin suppression. Thus, although there are some suggestions of changes in light sensitivity with aging in humans, the differences in response to light in healthy older versus young adults are not strong, and additional research in this area is needed to better understand whether changes in light sensitivity contribute to sleep and circadian rhythm timing changes with age.

Light Transmission

The changes in circadian responses to light that have been observed in some studies may be due to age-related changes in the pathway through the eye, along the retinohypothalamic tract (RHT), and/or within the SCN.[130] There is extensive evidence for changes in the transmission of light through the crystalline lens with age.[130–132] The aging lens accumulates yellow pigmentation, which selectively reduces transmission of short-wavelength light.[129,130,132] Although the exact relevance of this for humans living freely in environments where they can control ambient polychromatic lighting is not yet clear, a study of nearly 1000 Danish adults found that the age-related increase in yellowing of the lens was associated with greater reported sleep disturbances.[133]

There are also changes in the pupil with aging, with older adults having a smaller pupil than young adults. Daneault and colleagues[134] tested whether this affects response to monochromatic light exposure. They found that, although older adults had smaller pupils at dark-adapted baseline and at all light levels tested, the reduction in pupil size in response to light was not different between young and older subjects. Thus, available evidence suggests that light transmission through the lens is altered with age, specifically reducing transmission of short-wavelength light. Age-related changes in retinal function have also been reported in humans,[135,136] and there is a report that the number of intrinsically photosensitive retinal ganglion cells (ipRGCs) declines with age in rodless-coneless mice,[137] although the same group reported no change in responsiveness to light in the same type of older mice.[138]

Suprachiasmatic Nucleus

Although studies of human SCN function cannot be carried out, there is a general consensus based on animal studies that there are age-related changes in the SCN (reviewed, eg, in Ref.[139]). Studies carried out more than 2 decades ago demonstrated that the locomotor activity pattern of aged animals was much more consolidated after transplantation of fetal SCN, suggesting that some unknown factors that had declined with age had been reintroduced or improved.[140–143] There is strong evidence of altered patterns of electrical activity in the SCN of aged animals,[99–101] which is likely due to altered synchrony among SCN neurons, which leads to a reduced rhythm of multiunit activity.[102] Within individual SCN cells, changes in cell membrane properties that alter electrical activity of the cells have been demonstrated in older animals.[144] There is conflicting evidence about whether the size or cell number within the SCN is altered with age,[145–148] but there is general consensus that the aged SCN shows reductions in the number of cells expressing 2 major peptides, vasoactive intestinal polypeptide and arginine-vasopressin, in both animals and humans.[146–156]

Clock Gene Expression

There is some evidence from animal studies that clock gene expression is altered in aging, although not all studies are in agreement. One study found that expression of Per1 in response to an entraining light stimulus was reduced in aged hamsters, and this was associated with a significantly longer time to resynchronization.[157] That same study also found that the amplitude of Per1 and Per2 were not altered in older hamsters studied in constant darkness, but Bmal1 and Clock were altered in older hamsters. In a study of young and older mice, the amplitude of Per2 expression (but not expression of Per1, Clock, or Cry) was found to be reduced in the SCN of older mice.[158] A more comprehensive study of clock gene expression in young and older mice found age-related differences in expression of Per2, Bmal1, Rev-erbα, Dbp, and Dec1 in the SCN of the older mice.[159] Thus, even with the limited number of studies thus far, there is evidence that the molecular clockwork itself may be altered in aging, although much more research in this area remains to be done.

Circadian Rhythm Sleep-Wake Disorders

Older adults in general sleep and wake at earlier times than do young adults, and in general older adults are more likely to report advanced sleep-wake phase disorder than are young adults.[160,161] These patients report inability to stay awake in the evening and earlier than desired wake time. Delayed sleep-wake phase disorder and non-24-hour sleep-wake disorder show the reverse trend, with far fewer older adults complaining of sleep timing that is later than desired.[161] There is evidence that older adults are more prone to shift work disorder[162–167] and jet lag disorder, and this has been hypothesized to be due to a greater inability to sleep at an adverse biological time with age[11,28,30,31,46] and/or a reduced ability to phase shift with age. In addition to those circadian rhythm sleep disorders that affect community-dwelling older adults, there is evidence that institutionalized older adults and older adults with neurodegenerative diseases such as Alzheimer disease have high rates of irregular sleep-wake rhythm disorder.[168–172] This disorder is characterized by extremely irregular and fragmented sleep-wake patterns, and the disrupted sleep-wake rhythms are associated with very little bright light exposure,[173–175] which may potentially provide feedback and exacerbate the disrupted sleep patterns.[175] Interventions in which ambient lighting is increased have been tested in institutionalized settings and in some cases have been demonstrated to improve sleep-wake consolidation.[176–178]

SUMMARY

The most prominent age-related change in biological timing in humans is the shift of sleep to earlier hours. Why this occurs is still largely unknown. There is evidence for age-related changes in many aspects of circadian rhythmicity, including the transcriptional-translational feedback loops involved in circadian rhythm generation, the neuroanatomical structures, the transmission and responsiveness to light, and the timing and amplitude of output rhythms.

ACKNOWLEDGMENTS

The authors wish to thank J. Hong for assistance with the article.

REFERENCES

1. Duffy JF, Dijk DJ, Klerman EB, et al. Later endogenous circadian temperature nadir relative to an earlier wake time in older people. Am J Physiol 1998;275:R1478–87.

2. Gerard P, Collins KJ, Dore C, et al. Subjective characteristics of sleep in the elderly. Age Ageing 1978; 7:55–9.

3. Miles LE, Dement WC. Sleep and aging. Sleep 1980;3:119–220.

4. Monk TH, Reynolds CF III, Buysse DJ, et al. Circadian characteristics of healthy 80-year-olds and their relationship to objectively recorded sleep. J Gerontol 1991;46:M171–5.

5. Tune GS. The influence of age and temperament on the adult human sleep-wakefulness pattern. Br J Psychol 1969;60:431–41.

6. Van Coevorden A, Mockel J, Laurent E, et al. Neuroendocrine rhythms and sleep in aging men. Am J Physiol 1991;260:E651–61.

7. Van Someren EJ. Circadian and sleep disturbances in the elderly. Exp Gerontol 2000;35: 1229–37.

8. Foley DJ, Monjan AA, Brown SL, et al. Sleep complaints among elderly persons: an epidemiologic study of three communities. Sleep 1995;18: 425–32.

9. Mant A, Eyland EA. Sleep patterns and problems in elderly general practice attenders: an Australian survey. Community Health Stud 1988;12:192–9.

10. McGhie A, Russell SM. The subjective assessment of normal sleep patterns. J Ment Sci 1962;108:642–54.

11. Dijk DJ, Duffy JF, Czeisler CA. Age-related increase in awakenings: impaired consolidation of non-REM sleep at all circadian phases. Sleep 2001;24:565–77.

12. Bixler EO, Kales A, Jacoby JA, et al. Nocturnal sleep and wakefulness: effects of age and sex in normal sleepers. Int J Neurosci 1984;23:33–42.

13. Blois R, Feinberg I, Gaillard JM, et al. Sleep in normal and pathological aging. Experientia 1983; 39:551–8.

14. Brezinova V. The number and duration of the episodes of the various EEG stages of sleep in young and older people. Electroencephalogr Clin Neurophysiol 1975;39:273–8.

15. Dijk DJ, Beersma DGM, van den Hoofdakker RH. All night spectral analysis of EEG sleep in young adult and middle-aged male subjects. Neurobiol Aging 1989;10:677–82.

16. Ehlers CL, Kupfer DJ. Effects of age on delta and REM sleep parameters. Electroencephalogr Clin Neurophysiol 1989;72:118–25.

17. Feinberg I. Changes in sleep cycle patterns with age. J Psychiatr Res 1974;10:283–306.

18. Foret J, Webb WB. Evolution de l'organisation temporelle des stades de sommeil chez l'homme de 20 a 70 ans. Rev Electroencephalogr Neurophysiol Clin 1980;10:171–6.

19. Hayashi Y, Endo S. All-night sleep polygraphic recordings of healthy aged persons: REM and slow-wave sleep. Sleep 1982;5:277–83.

20. Kahn E, Fisher C. The sleep characteristics of the normal aged male. J Nerv Ment Dis 1969;148: 477–94.

21. Prinz PN. Sleep patterns in the healthy aged: relationship with intellectual function. J Gerontol 1977; 32:179–86.

22. Prinz PN, Vitiello MV, Raskind MA, et al. Geriatrics: sleep disorders and aging. N Engl J Med 1990; 323:520–6.

23. Reynolds CF III, Kupfer DJ, Taska LS, et al. Sleep of healthy seniors: a revisit. Sleep 1985;8:20–9.

24. Webb WB. The measurement and characteristics of sleep in older persons. Neurobiol Aging 1982; 3:311–9.

25. Webb WB, Campbell SS. Awakenings and the return to sleep in an older population. Sleep 1980; 3:41–6.

26. Bliwise DL. Sleep in normal aging and dementia. Sleep 1993;16:40–81.

27. Prinz PN. Sleep and sleep disorders in older adults. J Clin Neurophysiol 1995;12:139–46.

28. Dijk DJ, Duffy JF, Riel E, et al. Ageing and the circadian and homeostatic regulation of human sleep during forced desynchrony of rest, melatonin and temperature rhythms. J Physiol (Lond) 1999; 516(2):611–27.

29. Dijk DJ, Kelly TK, Riel E, et al. Altered homeostatic delta EEG response to sleep loss in older people? Sleep 1999;22:S226.

30. Dijk DJ, Duffy JF. Circadian regulation of human sleep and age-related changes in its timing, consolidation and EEG characteristics. Ann Med 1999;31:130–40.

31. Dijk DJ, Duffy JF, Czeisler CA. Contribution of circadian physiology and sleep homeostasis to age-related changes in human sleep. Chronobiol Int 2000;17:285–311.

32. Morgan K, Dallosso H, Ebrahim S, et al. Characteristics of subjective insomnia in the elderly living at home. Age Ageing 1988;17:1–7.

33. Executive Summary of the 2003 Sleep in America poll. Washington, DC: National Sleep Foundation; 2003.

34. Ohayon MM, Caulet M, Guilleminault C. How a general population perceives its sleep and how this relates to the complaint of insomnia. Sleep 1997;20:715–23.

35. McCurry SM, Ancoli-Israel S. Sleep dysfunction in Alzheimer's disease and other dementias. Curr Treat Options Neurol 2003;5:261–72.

36. Ehlers CL, Kupfer DJ. Slow-wave sleep: do young adult men and women age differently? J Sleep Res 1997;6:211–5.

37. Haimov I, Lavie P. Circadian characteristics of sleep propensity function in healthy elderly: a comparison with young adults. Sleep 1997;20:294–300.

38. Carrier J, Frenette S, Montplaisir J, et al. Effects of periodic leg movements during sleep in

middle-aged subjects without sleep complaints. Mov Disord 2005;20:1127–32.

39. Carrier J, Monk TH, Buysse DJ, et al. Sleep and morningness-eveningness in the 'middle' years of life (20-59 y). J Sleep Res 1997;6:230–7.

40. Ohayon MM, Carskadon MA, Guilleminault C, et al. Meta-analysis of quantitative sleep parameters from childhood to old age in healthy individuals: developing normative sleep values across the human lifespan. Sleep 2004;27:1255–73.

41. Borbély AA. A two process model of sleep regulation. Hum Neurobiol 1982;1:195–204.

42. Dijk DJ, Czeisler CA. Contribution of the circadian pacemaker and the sleep homeostat to sleep propensity, sleep structure, electroencephalographic slow waves, and sleep spindle activity in humans. J Neurosci 1995;15:3526–38.

43. Czeisler CA, Weitzman ED, Moore-Ede MC, et al. Human sleep: its duration and organization depend on its circadian phase. Science 1980; 210:1264–7.

44. Strogatz SH, Kronauer RE, Czeisler CA. Circadian regulation dominates homeostatic control of sleep length and prior wake length in humans. Sleep 1986;9:353–64.

45. Carskadon MA, Dement WC, Mitler MM, et al. Guidelines for the multiple sleep latency test (MSLT): a standard measure of sleepiness. Sleep 1986;9:519–24.

46. Hughes R, Sack RL, Lewy AJ. The role of melatonin and circadian phase in age-related sleep-maintenance insomnia: assessment in a clinical trial of melatonin replacement. Sleep 1998;21:52–68.

47. Fookson JE, Kronauer RE, Weitzman ED, et al. Induction of insomnia on a non-24 hour sleep-wake schedule. Sleep Res 1984;13:220.

48. Orth DN, Island DP. Light synchronization of the circadian rhythm in plasma cortisol (17-OHCS) concentration in man. J Clin Endocrinol Metab 1969;29:479–86.

49. Campbell SS, Dawson D. Aging young sleep: a test of the phase advance hypothesis of sleep disturbance in the elderly. Sleep Res 1991;20:447.

50. Ozaki S, Uchiyama M, Shirakawa S, et al. Prolonged interval from body temperature nadir to sleep offset in patients with delayed sleep phase syndrome. Sleep 1996;19:36–40.

51. Campbell SS, Dawson D, Anderson MW. Alleviation of sleep maintenance insomnia with timed exposure to bright light. J Am Geriatr Soc 1993;41:829–36.

52. Lavie P. Ultrashort sleep-waking schedule III. 'Gates' and 'forbidden zones' for sleep. Electroencephalogr Clin Neurophysiol 1986;63:414–25.

53. Strogatz SH, Kronauer RE, Czeisler CA. Circadian pacemaker interferes with sleep onset at specific times each day: role in insomnia. Am J Physiol 1987;253:R172–8.

54. Dijk DJ, Czeisler CA. Paradoxical timing of the circadian rhythm of sleep propensity serves to consolidate sleep and wakefulness in humans. Neurosci Lett 1994;166:63–8.

55. Dijk DJ, Duffy JF, Czeisler CA. Circadian and sleep/wake dependent aspects of subjective alertness and cognitive performance. J Sleep Res 1992;1: 112–7.

56. Boivin DB, Czeisler CA, Dijk DJ, et al. Complex interaction of the sleep-wake cycle and circadian phase modulates mood in healthy subjects. Arch Gen Psychiatry 1997;54:145–52.

57. Cajochen C, Wyatt JK, Czeisler CA, et al. Separation of circadian and wake duration-dependent modulation of EEG activation during wakefulness. Neurosci 2002;114:1047–60.

58. Duffy JF, Dijk DJ, Czeisler CA. Circadian and homeostatic modulation of cognitive throughput in older subjects. Sleep 1998;21:301.

59. Johnson MP, Duffy JF, Dijk DJ, et al. Short-term memory, alertness and performance: a reappraisal of their relationship to body temperature. J Sleep Res 1992;1:24–9.

60. Silva EJ, Wang W, Ronda JM, et al. Circadian and wake-dependent influences on subjective sleepiness, cognitive throughput, and reaction time performance in older and young adults. Sleep 2010; 33:481–90.

61. Lee JH, Wang W, Silva EJ, et al. Neurobehavioral performance in young adults living on a 28-h day for 6 weeks. Sleep 2009;32:905–13.

62. Czeisler CA, Duffy JF, Shanahan TL, et al. Stability, precision, and near-24-hour period of the human circadian pacemaker. Science 1999;284: 2177–81.

63. Campbell SS, Dawson D, Zulley J. When the human circadian system is caught napping: evidence for endogenous rhythms close to 24 hours. Sleep 1993;16:638–40.

64. Middleton B, Arendt J, Stone BM. Human circadian rhythms in constant dim light (8 lux) with knowledge of clock time. J Sleep Res 1996;5:69–76.

65. Hiddinga AE, Beersma DGM, van den Hoofdakker RH. Endogenous and exogenous components in the circadian variation of core body temperature in humans. J Sleep Res 1997;6:156–63.

66. Carskadon MA, Labyak SE, Acebo C, et al. Intrinsic circadian period of adolescent humans measured in conditions of forced desynchrony. Neurosci Lett 1999;260:129–32.

67. Smith MR, Burgess HJ, Fogg LF, et al. Racial differences in the human endogenous circadian period. PLoS One 2009;4:e6014.

68. Duffy JF, Cain SW, Chang AM, et al. Sex difference in the near-24-hour intrinsic period of the human circadian timing system. Proc Natl Acad Sci U S A 2011;108:15602–8.

69. Czeisler CA, Kronauer RE, Allan JS, et al. Bright light induction of strong (type 0) resetting of the human circadian pacemaker. Science 1989;244: 1328–33.

70. Khalsa SBS, Jewett ME, Cajochen C, et al. A phase response curve to single bright light pulses in human subjects. J Physiol (Lond) 2003;549:945–52.

71. Wright KP Jr, Gronfier C, Duffy JF, et al. Intrinsic period and light intensity determine the phase relationship between melatonin and sleep in humans. J Biol Rhythms 2005;20:168–77.

72. Mills JN, Minors DS, Waterhouse JM. Adaptation to abrupt time shifts of the oscillator[s] controlling human circadian rhythms. J Physiol (Lond) 1978;285: 455–70.

73. Duffy JF, Dijk DJ. Getting through to circadian oscillators: why use constant routines? J Biol Rhythms 2002;17:4–13.

74. Monk TH, Buysse DJ, Reynolds CF III, et al. Circadian temperature rhythms of older people. Exp Gerontol 1995;30:455–74.

75. Lieberman HR, Wurtman JJ, Teicher MH. Circadian rhythms of activity in healthy young and elderly humans. Neurobiol Aging 1989;10:259–65.

76. Weitzman ED, Moline ML, Czeisler CA, et al. Chronobiology of aging: temperature, sleep-wake rhythms and entrainment. Neurobiol Aging 1982; 3:299–309.

77. Touitou Y, Sulon J, Bogdan A, et al. Adrenal circadian system in young and elderly human subjects: a comparative study. J Endocrinol 1982;93:201–10.

78. Sherman B, Wysham C, Pfohl B. Age-related changes in the circadian rhythm of plasma cortisol in man. J Clin Endocrinol Metab 1985;61:439–43.

79. Sharma M, Palacios-Bois J, Schwartz G, et al. Circadian rhythms of melatonin and cortisol in aging. Biol Psychiatry 1989;25:305–19.

80. Czeisler CA, Dumont M, Duffy JF, et al. Association of sleep-wake habits in older people with changes in output of circadian pacemaker. Lancet 1992; 340:933–6.

81. Carrier J, Monk TH, Reynolds CF III, et al. Are age differences in sleep due to phase differences in the output of the circadian timing system? Chronobiol Int 1999;16:79–91.

82. Carrier J, Paquet J, Morettini J, et al. Phase advance of sleep and temperature circadian rhythms in the middle years of life in humans. Neurosci Lett 2002;320:1–4.

83. Kim SJ, Benloucif S, Reid KJ, et al. Phase-shifting response to light in older adults. J Physiol 2014; 592:189–202.

84. Duffy JF, Zeitzer JM, Rimmer DW, et al. Peak of circadian melatonin rhythm occurs later within the sleep of older subjects. Am J Physiol 2002;282: E297–303.

85. Lewy AJ, Bauer VK, Singer CM, et al. Later circadian phase of plasma melatonin relative to usual waketime in older subjects. Sleep 2000; 23:A188–9.

86. Tozawa T, Mishima K, Satoh K, et al. Stability of sleep timing against the melatonin secretion rhythm with advancing age: clinical implications. J Clin Endocrinol Metab 2003;88:4689–95.

87. Van Cauter E, Leproult R, Kupfer DJ. Effects of gender and age on the levels and circadian rhythmicity of plasma cortisol. J Clin Endocrinol Metab 1996;81:2468–73.

88. Kripke DF, Elliott JA, Youngstedt SD, et al. Circadian phase response curves to light in older and young women and men. J Circadian Rhythms 2007;5:4.

89. Pittendrigh CS, Daan S. A functional analysis of circadian pacemakers in nocturnal rodents. IV. Entrainment: pacemaker as clock. J Comp Physiol [A] 1976;106:291–331.

90. Zee PC, Rosenberg RS, Turek FW. Effects of aging on entrainment and rate of resynchronization of circadian locomotor activity. Am J Physiol 1992; 263:R1099–103.

91. Scarbrough K, Losee-Olson S, Wallen EP, et al. Aging and photoperiod affect entrainment and quantitative aspects of locomotor behavior in Syrian hamsters. Am J Physiol 1997;272:R1219–25.

92. Valentinuzzi VS, Scarbrough K, Takahashi JS, et al. Effects of aging on the circadian rhythm of wheel-running activity in C57BL/6 mice. Am J Physiol 1997;273:R1957–64.

93. Buysse DJ, Monk TH, Carrier J, et al. Circadian patterns of sleep, sleepiness, and performance in older and younger adults. Sleep 2005;28:1365–76.

94. Münch M, Knoblauch V, Blatter K, et al. Age-related attenuation of the evening circadian arousal signal in humans. Neurobiol Aging 2005;26:1307–19.

95. Yoon IY, Kripke DF, Elliott JA, et al. Age-related changes of circadian rhythms and sleep-wake cycles. J Am Geriatr Soc 2003;51:1085–91.

96. Davis FC, Viswanathan N. Stability of circadian timing with age in Syrian hamsters. Am J Physiol 1998;275:R960–8.

97. Duffy JF, Viswanathan N, Davis FC. Free-running circadian period does not shorten with age in female Syrian hamsters. Neurosci Lett 1999;271:77–80.

98. Penev P, Zee P, Turek FW. Quantitative analysis of the age-related fragmentation of hamster 24-h activity rhythms. Am J Physiol 1997;273:R2132–7.

99. Satinoff E, Li H, Tcheng TK, et al. Do the suprachiasmatic nuclei oscillate in old rats as they do in young ones? Am J Physiol 1993;265:R1216–22.

100. Watanabe A, Shibata S, Watanabe S. Circadian rhythm of spontaneous neuronal activity in the suprachiasmatic nucleus of old hamster in vitro. Brain Res 1995;695:237–9.

101. Nakamura TJ, Nakamura W, Yamazaki S, et al. Age-related decline in circadian output. J Neurosci 2011; 31:10201–5.

102. Farajnia S, Michel S, Deboer T, et al. Evidence for neuronal desynchrony in the aged suprachiasmatic nucleus clock. J Neurosci 2012;32:5891–9.

103. Carrier J, Monk TH, Buysse DJ, et al. Amplitude reduction of the circadian temperature and sleep rhythms in the elderly. Chronobiol Int 1996;13: 373–86.

104. Zeitzer JM, Daniels JE, Duffy JF, et al. Do plasma melatonin concentrations decline with age? Am J Med 1999;107:432–6.

105. Silva EJ, Cain SW, Munch MY, et al. Age-related differences in the effect of chronic sleep restriction on sleep quality. Sleep 2011;34:A24.

106. Cain SW, Silva EJ, Munch MY, et al. Chronic sleep restriction impairs reaction time performance more in young than in older subjects. Sleep 2010; 33:A85.

107. Zitting K-M, Cain SW, Munch MY, et al. Objective sleepiness in young and older adults during 3-weeks of chronic sleep restriction. J Sleep Res 2014;23:269.

108. Pittendrigh CS, Daan S. Circadian oscillations in rodents: a systematic increase of their frequency with age. Science 1974;186:548–50.

109. Morin LP. Age-related changes in hamster circadian period, entrainment, and rhythm splitting. J Biol Rhythms 1988;3:237–48.

110. Rosenberg RS, Zee PC, Turek FW. Phase response curves to light in young and old hamsters. Am J Physiol 1991;261:R491–5.

111. Kendall AR, Lewy AJ, Sack RL. Effects of aging on the intrinsic circadian period of totally blind humans. J Biol Rhythms 2001;16:87–95.

112. Duffy JF, Czeisler CA. Effect of light on human circadian physiology. Sleep Med Clin 2009;4: 165–77.

113. Kelly TL, Neri DF, Grill JT, et al. Nonentrained circadian rhythms of melatonin in submariners scheduled to an 18-hour day. J Biol Rhythms 1999;14: 190–6.

114. Orth DN, Besser GM, King PH, et al. Free-running circadian plasma cortisol rhythm in a blind human subject. Clin Endocrinol (Oxf) 1979;10:603–17.

115. Jean-Louis G, Kripke DF, Ancoli-Israel S, et al. Circadian sleep, illumination, and activity patterns in women: influences of aging and time reference. Physiol Behav 2000;68:347–52.

116. Guillemette J, Hébert M, Paquet J, et al. Natural bright light exposure in the summer and winter in subjects with and without complaints of seasonal mood variations. Biol Psychiatry 1998;44:622–8.

117. Cole RJ, Kripke DF, Wisbey J, et al. Seasonal variation in human illumination exposure at two different latitudes. J Biol Rhythms 1995;10:324–34.

118. Burgess HJ, Eastman CI. Early versus late bedtimes phase shift the human dim light melatonin rhythm despite a fixed morning lights on time. Neurosci Lett 2004;356:115–8.

119. Gooley JJ, Chamberlain K, Smith KA, et al. Exposure to room light before bedtime suppresses melatonin onset and shortens melatonin duration in humans. J Clin Endocrinol Metab 2011;96: E463–72.

120. Santhi N, Thorne HC, van der Veen DR, et al. The spectral composition of evening light and individual differences in the suppression of melatonin and delay of sleep in humans. J Pineal Res 2011; 53:47–59.

121. Chang AM, Aeschbach D, Duffy JF, et al. Evening use of light-emitting eReaders negatively affects sleep, circadian timing, and next-morning alertness. Proc Natl Acad Sci U S A 2015;112: 1232–7.

122. Scheuermaier K, Laffan AM, Duffy JF. Light exposure patterns in healthy older and young adults. J Biol Rhythms 2010;25:113–22.

123. Kawinska A, Dumont M, Selmaoui B, et al. Are modifications of melatonin circadian rhythm in the middle years of life related to habitual patterns of light exposure? J Biol Rhythms 2005;20:451–60.

124. Klerman EB, Duffy JF, Dijk DJ, et al. Circadian phase resetting in older people by ocular bright light exposure. J Investig Med 2001;49:30–40.

125. Benloucif S, Green K, L'Hermite-Balériaux M, et al. Responsiveness of the aging circadian clock to light. Neurobiol Aging 2006;27:1870–9.

126. Duffy JF, Zeitzer JM, Czeisler CA. Decreased sensitivity to phase-delaying effects of moderate intensity light in older subjects. Neurobiol Aging 2007;28:799–807.

127. Herljevic M, Middleton B, Thapan K, et al. Light-induced melatonin suppression: age-related reduction in response to short wavelength light. Exp Gerontol 2005;40:237–42.

128. Sletten TL, Revell VL, Middleton B, et al. Age-related changes in acute and phase-advancing responses to monochromatic light. J Biol Rhythms 2009;24:73–84.

129. Najjar RP, Chiquet C, Teikari P, et al. Aging of non-visual spectral sensitivity to light in humans: compensatory mechanisms? PLoS One 2014;9: e85837.

130. Brainard GC, Rollag MD, Hanifin JP. Photic regulation of melatonin in humans: ocular and neural signal transduction. J Biol Rhythms 1997;12:537–46.

131. Barker FM, Brainard GC, Dayhaw-Barker P. Transmittance of the human lens as a function of age. 1991. ARVO Annual Meeting Abstracts. Sarasota, FL, April 28–May 3, 1991.

132. Zhang Y, Brainard GC, Zee PC, et al. Effects of aging on lens transmittance and retinal input to the

suprachiasmatic nucleus in golden hamsters. Neurosci Lett 1998;258:167–70.

133. Kessel L, Siganos G, Jorgensen T, et al. Sleep disturbances are related to decreased transmission of blue light to the retina caused by lens yellowing. Sleep 2011;34:1215–9.

134. Daneault V, Vandewalle G, Hebert M, et al. Does pupil constriction under blue and green monochromatic light exposure change with age? J Biol Rhythms 2012;27:257–64.

135. Freund PR, Watson J, Gilmour GS, et al. Differential changes in retina function with normal aging in humans. Doc Ophthalmol 2011;122:177–90.

136. Gerth C, Garcia SM, Ma L, et al. Multifocal electroretinogram: age-related changes for different luminance levels. Graefes Arch Clin Exp Ophthalmol 2002;240:202–8.

137. Semo M, Lupi D, Peirson SN, et al. Light-induced c-fos in melanopsin retinal ganglion cells of young and aged rodless/coneless (rd/rd cl) mice. Eur J Neurosci 2003;18:3007–17.

138. Semo M, Peirson S, Lupi D, et al. Melanopsin retinal ganglion cells and the maintenance of circadian and pupillary responses to light in aged rodless/coneless (rd/rd cl) mice. Eur J Neurosci 2003;17:1793–801.

139. Gibson EM, Williams WP 3rd, Kriegsfeld LJ. Aging in the circadian system: considerations for health, disease prevention and longevity. Exp Gerontol 2009;44:51–6.

140. Cai A, Scarbrough K, Hinkle DA, et al. Fetal grafts containing suprachiasmatic nuclei restore the diurnal rhythm of CRH and POMC mRNA in aging rats. Am J Physiol 1997;273:R1764–70.

141. Hurd MW, Zimmer KA, Lehman MN, et al. Circadian locomotor rhythms in aged hamsters following suprachiasmatic transplant. Am J Physiol 1995;269: R958–68.

142. Viswanathan N, Davis FC. Suprachiasmatic nucleus grafts restore circadian function in aged hamsters. Brain Res 1995;686:10–6.

143. Van Reeth O, Zhang Y, Zee PC, et al. Grafting fetal suprachiasmatic nuclei in the hypothalamus of old hamsters restores responsiveness of the circadian clock to a phase shifting stimulus. Brain Res 1994; 643:338–42.

144. Farajnia S, Meijer JH, Michel S. Age-related changes in large-conductance calcium-activated potassium channels in mammalian circadian clock neurons. Neurobiol Aging 2015;36:2176–83.

145. Madeira MD, Sousa N, Santer RM, et al. Age and sex do not affect the volume, cell numbers, or cell size of the suprachiasmatic nucleus of the rat: an unbiased stereological study. J Comp Neurol 1995;361:585–601.

146. Roozendaal B, van Gool WA, Swaab DF, et al. Changes in vasopressin cells of the rat suprachiasmatic nucleus with aging. Brain Res 1987;409:259–64.

147. Swaab DF, Fliers E, Partiman TS. The suprachiasmatic nucleus of the human brain in relation to sex, age and senile dementia. Brain Res 1985;342:37–44.

148. Hofman MA, Swaab DF. Living by the clock: the circadian pacemaker in older people. Ageing Res Rev 2006;5:33–51.

149. Kawakami F, Okamura H, Tamada Y, et al. Loss of day-night differences in VIP mRNA levels in the suprachiasmatic nucleus of aged rats. Neurosci Lett 1997;222:99–102.

150. Chee CA, Roozendaal B, Swaab DF, et al. Vasoactive intestinal polypeptide neuron changes in the senile rat suprachiasmatic nucleus. Neurobiol Aging 1988;9:307–12.

151. Hofman MA, Fliers E, Goudsmit E, et al. Morphometric analysis of the suprachiasmatic and paraventricular nuclei in the human brain: sex differences and age-dependent changes. J Anat 1988;160:127–43.

152. Aujard F, Cayetanot F, Bentivoglio M, et al. Age-related effects on the biological clock and its behavioral output in a primate. Chronobiol Int 2006;23:451–60.

153. Wang JL, Lim AS, Chiang WY, et al. Suprachiasmatic neuron numbers and rest-activity circadian rhythms in older humans. Ann Neurol 2015;78: 317–22.

154. Duncan MJ, Herron JM, Hill SA. Aging selectively suppresses vasoactive intestinal peptide messenger RNA expression in the suprachiasmatic nucleus of the Syrian hamster. Brain Res Mol Brain Res 2001;87:196–203.

155. Zhou J-N, Hofman MA, Swaab DF. VIP neurons in the human SCN in relation to sex, age, and Alzheimer's disease. Neurobiol Aging 1995;16:571–6.

156. Krajnak K, Kashon ML, Rosewell KL, et al. Aging alters the rhythmic expression of vasoactive intestinal polypeptide mRNA but not arginine vasopressin mRNA in the suprachiasmatic nuclei of female rats. J Neurosci 1998;18:4767–74.

157. Kolker DE, Fukuyama H, Huang DS, et al. Aging alters circadian and light-induced expression of clock genes in golden hamsters. J Biol Rhythms 2003;18:159–69.

158. Weinert D, Weinert H, Schurov I, et al. Impaired expression of the mPer2 circadian clock gene in the suprachiasmatic nuclei of aging mice. Chronobiol Int 2001;18:559–65.

159. Bonaconsa M, Malpeli G, Montaruli A, et al. Differential modulation of clock gene expression in the suprachiasmatic nucleus, liver and heart of aged mice. Exp Gerontol 2014;55:70–9.

160. Schrader H, Bovim G, Sand T. The prevalence of delayed and advanced sleep phase syndromes. J Sleep Res 1993;2:51–5.

161. Sack RL, Auckley D, Auger RR, et al. Circadian rhythm sleep disorders: part II, advanced sleep phase disorder, delayed sleep phase disorder, free-running disorder, and irregular sleep-wake rhythm. An American Academy of Sleep Medicine review. Sleep 2007;30:1484–501.

162. Sack RL, Auckley D, Auger RR, et al. Circadian rhythm sleep disorders: part I, basic principles, shift work and jet lag disorders. An American Academy of Sleep Medicine review. Sleep 2007; 30:1460–83.

163. Ftouni S, Sletten TL, Barger LK, et al. Shift work disorder. In: Barkoukis T, Matheson JK, Ferber R, et al, editors. Therapy in sleep medicine. Amsterdam: Elsevier; 2011. p. 411–24.

164. Duffy JF. Shift work and aging: roles of sleep and circadian rhythms. Clin Occup Environ Med 2003; 3:311–32.

165. Härmä MI, Hakola T, Åkerstedt T, et al. Age and adjustment to night work. Occup Environ Med 1994;51:568–73.

166. Marquié JC, Foret J. Sleep, age, and shiftwork experience. J Sleep Res 1999;8:297–304.

167. Åkerstedt T, Torsvall L. Age, sleep and adjustment to shiftwork. In: Koella WP, editor. Sleep 1980. Basel (Switzerland): S. Karger; 1981. p. 190–5.

168. Zee PC, Vitiello MV. Circadian rhythm sleep disorder: irregular sleep wake rhythm type. Sleep Med Clin 2009;4:213–8.

169. Ancoli-Israel S, Parker L, Sinaee R, et al. Sleep fragmentation in patients from a nursing home. J Gerontol 1989;44:M18–21.

170. Mirmiran M, Swaab DF, Kok JH, et al. Circadian rhythms and the suprachiasmatic nucleus in perinatal development, aging and Alzheimer's disease. Prog Brain Res 1992;93:151–63.

171. Witting W, Kwa IH, Eikelenboom P, et al. Alterations in the circadian rest-activity rhythm in aging and Alzheimer's disease. Biol Psychiatry 1990;27: 563–72.

172. van Someren EJW, Hagebeuk EEO, Lijzenga C, et al. Circadian rest-activity rhythm disturbances in Alzheimer's disease. Biol Psychiatry 1996;40: 259–70.

173. Campbell SS, Kripke DF, Gillin JC, et al. Exposure to light in healthy elderly subjects and Alzheimer's patients. Physiol Behav 1988;42:141–4.

174. Ancoli-Israel S, Klauber MR, Jones DW, et al. Variations in circadian rhythms of activity, sleep, and light exposure related to dementia in nursing-home patients. Sleep 1997;20:18–23.

175. Shochat T, Martin J, Marler M, et al. Illumination levels in nursing home patients: effects on sleep and activity rhythms. J Sleep Res 2000;9:373–9.

176. Ancoli-Israel S, Gehrman P, Martin JL, et al. Increased light exposure consolidates sleep and strengthens circadian rhythms in severe Alzheimer's disease patients. Behav Sleep Med 2003;1:22–36.

177. van Someren EJW, Kessler A, Mirmiran M, et al. Indirect bright light improves circadian rest-activity rhythm disturbances in demented patients. Biol Psychiatry 1997;41:955–63.

178. Riemersma-van der Lek RF, Swaab DF, Twisk J, et al. Effect of bright light and melatonin on cognitive and noncognitive function in elderly residents of group care facilities: a randomized controlled trial. JAMA 2008;299:2642–55.

Effect of Light and Melatonin and Other Melatonin Receptor Agonists on Human Circadian Physiology

Jonathan S. Emens, MD[a,b], Helen J. Burgess, PhD[c],*

KEYWORDS

• Advance • Agonist • Circadian • Delay • Light • Melatonin

KEY POINTS

• Circadian timing has a profound influence on mental health, physical health, and health behaviors.
• Individual patients suspected of misaligned circadian rhythms can vary in their suitability for light, melatonin, and other melatonin receptor agonist treatment.
• Prescribing a relatively consistent light/dark cycle is often the first step in treatment.
• Key features of light treatment to consider include timing, intensity, duration, color, light avoidance, and choosing a light device to best accommodate patient motivation for treatment.
• Key features of exogenous melatonin and other melatonin receptor agonist treatments to consider include timing, dose, fast or slow release formulations, and purity.

INTRODUCTION

Multiple varieties of light devices and multiple formulations of exogenous melatonin are commercially available without prescription in the United States. Light devices are most commonly used by patients with seasonal affective disorder, who represent approximately 1% to 2% of the North American general population.[1] Similarly, approximately 2% of US adults use exogenous melatonin, most typically as a sleep aid.[2,3] There are also several melatonin receptor agonist formulations available via prescription in various countries around the world.

Light, melatonin, and other melatonin receptor agonists can significantly impact circadian ("body clock") physiology, particularly the *timing* of circadian rhythms. Circadian timing in turn has a widespread and profound influence on mental and physical health (eg, Refs.[4–6]). For example, there are projections from the central circadian clock to peripheral tissues,[7,8] and the circadian clock has a direct influence on sleep[9] and inflammatory processes.[10] The central circadian clock also influences circadian clocks in peripheral systems.[11] The focus of this review was on the use of light, melatonin, and other melatonin receptor agonists to shift central circadian timing in patients in whom misaligned biological rhythms are thought to play a role, and the practical issues surrounding their use. Light can also suppress melatonin[12] and increase alertness,[13]

Disclosure Statement: The authors have nothing to disclose.
[a] Department of Hospital and Specialty Medicine, Portland VA Medical Center, 3710 SW US Veterans Hospital Road, P3-PULM, Portland, OR 97239, USA; [b] Departments of Psychiatry and Medicine, Oregon Health & Science University, 3181 SW Sam Jackson Park Road, Portland, OR 97239, USA; [c] Biological Rhythms Research Laboratory, Department of Behavioral Sciences, Rush University Medical Center, 1645 West Jackson Boulevard, Suite 425, Chicago, IL 60612, USA
* Corresponding author.
E-mail address: Helen_J_Burgess@rush.edu

Sleep Med Clin 10 (2015) 435–453
http://dx.doi.org/10.1016/j.jsmc.2015.08.001
1556-407X/15/$ – see front matter © 2015 Elsevier Inc. All rights reserved.

and exogenous melatonin can increase circulating levels of melatonin,[14] but here we restrict our focus to circadian phase shifting, as this is most often the aim of light and melatonin treatment. We intend for this review to complement rather than replace clinical recommendations on the use of light, melatonin, and other melatonin receptor agonists to treat circadian rhythm sleep disorders (Ref.[15]), depression (eg, Refs.[16,17]), and/or insomnia (eg, Ref.[18]). We provide a brief review of the human circadian system, followed by a summary of the patient characteristics and safety issues to consider before recommending light treatment, melatonin, or other melatonin receptor agonists to patients. We then review the characteristics of light that are relevant to circadian physiology, and practical aspects of light treatment and conversely, light avoidance. The important features of exogenous melatonin and other melatonin receptor agonists are then described, followed by practical aspects of melatonin treatment and, briefly, how melatonin can be combined with light treatment to increase shifts in circadian timing. We end with a consideration of how to evaluate patient outcomes after treatment.

THE CENTRAL CIRCADIAN SYSTEM

The central circadian system can be conceptualized as having 3 components: (1) input pathways that provide signals to synchronize the endogenous central clock to the external environment, (2) the central clock, which generates the rhythms, and (3) output pathways or rhythms that convey the central clock signal to other regulatory systems in the brain and body (**Fig. 1**). In terms of input pathways, the strongest resetting agent is light. Light is captured by the 5 retinal photoreceptors (rods, blue cones, green cones, red cones, and the intrinsically photosensitive retinal ganglion cells [ipRGCs]) and the signal is transmitted to the central circadian clock.[19] Other "nonphotic" stimuli, such as exogenous melatonin, can also be used to shift circadian timing. Here we refer to *exogenous melatonin* as melatonin that people typically ingest, after which it enters the circulation and is believed to shift circadian timing by binding to melatonin receptors on the central clock.[20]

The central circadian clock is located in the suprachiasmatic nuclei (SCN) in the hypothalamus.[21] More than 70% of humans have an endogenous period greater than 24 hours (on average ~24.2 hours).[22,23] Thus, for most humans, their internal body clock takes more than 24 hours to complete 1 cycle, meaning that they have an endogenous tendency to drift later ("phase delay") each day. This is perhaps most commonly seen in the later sleep times that often occur on the weekend or work-free days.[24] A gradual later drift in circadian timing is also seen in totally blind individuals, as light does not reach their internal circadian clock.[25] Thus, daily input signals are required to shift the clock earlier ("phase advance") to synchronize the clock's timing to the external 24-hour day.

The output circadian rhythm often measured to infer the timing of the central circadian clock in humans is the endogenous melatonin rhythm. We use the term *endogenous melatonin* to refer to internally produced melatonin. The endogenous melatonin rhythm is believed to accurately represent the timing of the central circadian clock, as the secretion of melatonin from the pineal gland

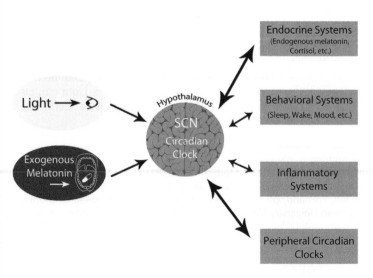

Fig. 1. The 3 components of the circadian system: (1) input pathways such as light and exogenous melatonin, which provide timing signals to the central circadian clock; (2) the central clock, SCN in the hypothalamus, which generates the rhythms; and (3) the output rhythms, which include endogenous melatonin and molecular peripheral circadian clocks contained in most tissues. Many of these output rhythms can feedback to the central circadian clock.

is controlled by the SCN.[26] Endogenous melatonin also likely feeds back to bind to the central clock and reinforces circadian timing.[27] Currently, the most reliable marker of circadian timing is the dim light melatonin onset (DLMO),[28] which is the time when endogenous melatonin levels begin to rise in dim light approximately 2 to 3 hours before habitual bedtime[29] (**Fig. 2**). Endogenous melatonin must be measured in dim light, as light suppresses melatonin.[12,30] The DLMO is most easily assessed via half-hourly or hourly saliva samples collected in the approximately 6 hours or so before habitual bedtime, which are later assayed for melatonin concentration.[31]

In addition to the endogenous melatonin rhythm, it is important to note that the central circadian clock drives a whole host of other output rhythms, and impacts multiple other systems including, but not limited to, endocrine systems,[32] metabolism,[33] inflammation,[10] mood,[6,34,35] and behaviors, including sleep.[36] Indeed, whether a direct or indirect influence, mistiming of circadian rhythms is also associated with an increase in negative health behaviors, such as the excessive consumption of alcohol, caffeine, and nicotine[37] and is also associated with unhealthy dietary habits.[38] It has been hypothesized that mistimed circadian rhythms play a role in mood disorders as well.[35,39] As the importance of circadian timing to mental and physical health is increasingly recognized, we anticipate light and/or exogenous melatonin will be increasingly used as adjunctive treatments to other therapies. Light treatment in particular, as a nonpharmacological therapy, is likely to be attractive to many patients.

PATIENT EVALUATION OVERVIEW AND SAFETY CONSIDERATIONS

When considering light or exogenous melatonin treatment, the clinician should first address whether the etiology of the presenting signs and/or symptoms may be at least partly due to a mistiming of the circadian system (**Fig. 3**). In the case of circadian rhythm sleep disorders, this is fairly straightforward, as the etiology is assumed to rest with a misalignment between the timing of the clock and the desired timing of sleep and wakefulness. However, in depression and insomnia, as well as circadian rhythm sleep disorders, it can often be difficult in practice to determine whether the etiology of a patient's complaint is circadian in nature. For example, sleep-onset insomnia can result from a circadian phase delay but might also be the direct result of medical or psychiatric illness, environmental disturbances, substances, or a host of other factors. The picture is further complicated because a shift in the timing of the clock might be the result of another disorder (eg, back pain might cause early morning awakening that in turn results in exposure to phase-advancing morning light). In this way, circadian resetting might be a

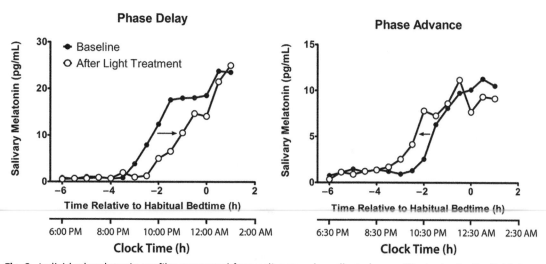

Fig. 2. Individual melatonin profiles generated from saliva samples collected every 30 minutes in dim light. Baseline dim light melatonin profiles are shown in black circles. In both individuals, the DLMO occurs approximately 3.0 to 3.5 hours before habitual bedtime. Note that the clock time of the DLMOs varies according to the clock time of habitual bedtime in each individual. On the left, the dim light melatonin profile shifts later in clock time, after exposure to evening bright light (phase delay). On the right the dim light melatonin profile shifts earlier in clock time, after exposure to morning bright light (phase advance).

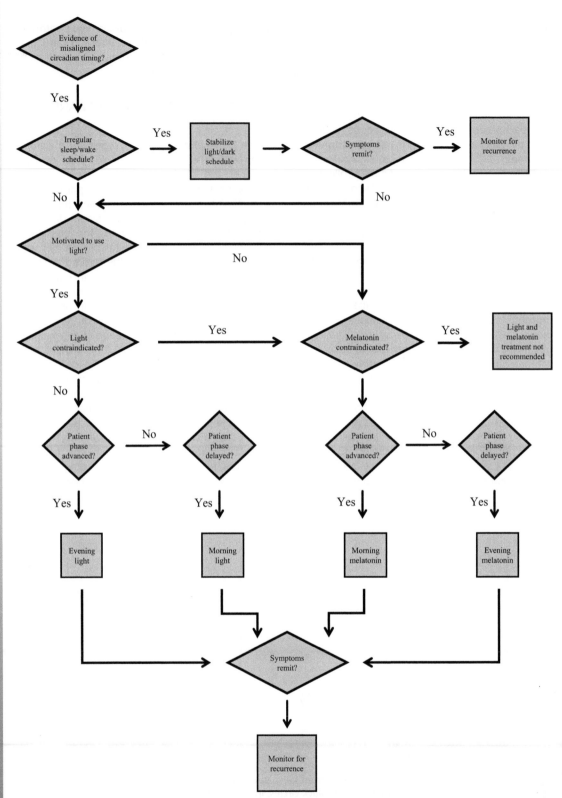

Fig. 3. A flow diagram illustrating an example of clinical questions that should be asked when considering light and melatonin treatment. Note that as discussed in the text, light and melatonin can be used in combination to augment circadian phase advances. It has not yet been determined if the addition of melatonin to light can augment circadian phase delays.

perpetuating factor as opposed to a precipitating one. Nonetheless, symptoms of sleep-onset insomnia and morning hypersomnolence or fatigue are at least suggestive of a phase delay in circadian timing, whereas symptoms of late afternoon/early evening hypersomnolence or fatigue and early morning awakening are suggestive of a phase advance in circadian timing. Evaluation of symptoms of depression as they relate to the circadian system are beyond the scope of this review, but suffice to say that both phase advances and phase delays have been hypothesized to play a role.[17,34]

Another important consideration is the *consistency* of the patient's light/dark schedule, which is largely determined by the consistency of their sleep/wake schedule. In nature, the small variability in the timing of light and darkness from day to day (on the order of minutes) is easily accommodated by the circadian system. However, under conditions of artificial light, it is not uncommon to see variation in the light/dark cycle on the order of hours. This variability, most often greatest between work days and work-free days, can cause a misalignment between the timing of the central circadian clock and the desired timing of sleep and wakefulness ("social jet-lag").[37] Moreover, this variability in the light/dark cycle can confound the clinician's efforts to reset the circadian pacemaker, as the prescribed resetting "signal" risks being partially lost in the "noise" of a variable light/dark schedule. For this reason, in patients with variable sleep/wake schedules, such as those with sleep onset and/or wake times that vary, for example, by more than 3 hours in a week, we recommend either first, or in conjunction with light and/or exogenous melatonin treatment, working with the patient to try to reduce the variability in sleep/wake timing and also the variability in light/dark timing.

Motivation for treatment also should be assessed, as this can be a significant barrier to the use of light given the time involved and potential limitations on other activities during light therapy. The potential contraindications also should be considered (see the bulleted items that follow). These contraindications are not based on large randomized clinical trials, but rather represent a cautious approach. Bright light is associated with some side effects, the most common being headache, eyestrain, nausea, and agitation,[40] but often these side effects spontaneously remit,[40,41] and subjects rarely discontinue due to side effects.[41] Bright light is generally considered safe with no changes in extensive ophthalmologic examination observed after up to 6 years of daily use (in fall and winter

months in patients with seasonal affective disorder).[42] A rare but serious side effect of bright light therapy is mania in bipolar patients who overexpose themselves to the light.[40,41] In our clinical practice and clinical trials, no significant side effects or adverse events due to bright light treatment have occurred.

Potential contraindications to bright light treatment

- Existing eye disease
- Migraine headaches (if elicited by light)
- Phototoxic medication use
- History of mania

Side effects, besides sleepiness, are infrequent with exogenous melatonin, but increased depressive symptoms, headaches, hypertension and hypotension, and gastrointestinal upset have been associated with exogenous melatonin administration.[43,44] There have been concerns about potential developmental effects in children (eg, effects on growth hormone[45]), although one study found no effects on pubertal development.[46] Nonetheless, it is prudent to exercise caution in the administration of melatonin to prepubertal children unless the risk-benefit analysis strongly favors treatment (eg, in children with significant developmental delay or children with non–24-hour sleep-wake schedule disorder). Although lower *endogenous* melatonin levels have been shown to be associated with increased risk of type 2 diabetes,[47] one study found that exogenous melatonin (5 mg) when administered with food acutely impaired glucose tolerance.[48] More research investigating the effects of exogenous melatonin on glucose metabolism is required. It should be noted here that melatonin is not regulated by the Food and Drug Administration (FDA) and we discuss issues of purity later in this article.

Several melatonin agonists or prescription melatonin formulations are discussed later in this article, and they carry their own potential side-effect profiles, including increased risk of liver injury with agomelatine[49,50]; headache, elevated liver enzymes, cardiac conduction changes, upper respiratory and urinary tract infections, and nightmares for tasimelteon[51]; and headache, sleepiness, upper respiratory tract infections, gastrointestinal upset, dizziness, and dysmenorrheal for ramelteon.[52] Circadin is an extended release formulation of melatonin and has a similar side-effect profile to melatonin.[53]

Potential contraindications to exogenous melatonin treatment
• History of excessive sedation with melatonin use, especially with driving or operating equipment
• Pregnancy or nursing or seeking to become pregnant
• Children (except those with significant neuro-developmental delay or non–24-hour disorder)[45,46]
• Warfarin therapy[43]
• Epilepsy[43,54]

USING LIGHT TO SHIFT CIRCADIAN TIMING
Timing of Light

One of the most complicated aspects of light treatment is that the timing of light treatment is critical to the resulting shift in circadian timing. Indeed, it is possible to generate completely opposite shifts in circadian timing with precisely the same light, depending solely on when the light is administered *relative to the timing of the internal circadian clock*. To help assist in predicting what the effect of light treatment is likely to have on circadian timing, mathematical functions called "phase response curves" (PRCs) have been developed (eg, Ref.[55]). PRCs can be understood by imagining your participation in a laboratory experiment. You are first asked to maintain a consistent sleep/wake schedule with an 8-hour sleep opportunity for a week or more at home to stabilize your circadian timing. At the end of this baseline week, you arrive at the laboratory in the afternoon, are seated in dim light and every 30 minutes provide a saliva sample up until or even past your usual bedtime. Then, you sit in front of a light box for an hour, before sleeping in the laboratory. You awake the next morning and remain in the laboratory until later that afternoon you repeat the dim light saliva collection. The saliva samples are later assayed for melatonin and your individual DLMO (see **Fig. 2**) is calculated for each saliva collection session. Your first baseline DLMO is then compared with your second post–light treatment DLMO. The phase shift in the DLMO is plotted on a y-axis: positive number if the DLMO shifted earlier in time after light treatment (phase advance), negative number if the DLMO shifted later in time after light treatment (phase delay), or on zero line if no shift in DLMO. On the x-axis, the data point is plotted as the start of light treatment *relative to your baseline DLMO*; in this case it would probably be several hours after your baseline DLMO. This

experiment is then repeated again and again, until there are many data points covering the breadth of the x-axis, reflecting that the light treatment was administered at all different circadian (DLMO) times. The data points are then curve fit with the resulting mathematical function revealing what phase shifts are likely to result when light is administered at different times relative to the DLMO. There are a variety of experimental protocols used to construct a PRC, but all follow the same basic pattern of assessment of circadian phase, exposure to a resetting stimulus, and then reassessment of circadian phase.

There are several limitations to PRCs that are important to keep in mind. First, PRCs represent a global average across the individuals who participated in the research protocol that generated the PRC. These individuals may have distinct individual differences in their response to the resetting stimulus, for example, light. Thus, the average PRC is unlikely to accurately predict the effect of light treatment in an individual patient. Second, the protocols used to generate PRCs often include the unusual timing or shifting of sleep/dark, which may not generalize to the nocturnal sleep timing of many patients. Accordingly, we may not be as sensitive to light in the middle of day as the light PRC suggests us to be. Indeed, studies of either bright light or darkness in the afternoon found no changes in circadian timing.[56,57] Third, most PRCs are referenced to the timing of the DLMO. To date, the DLMO is not commonly measured in the clinic, although validated home procedures may become part of standard clinical practice in the future.[58] Currently, without access to the timing of the DLMO, the next best estimate of the PRC is to consider it relative to habitual sleep timing, as the DLMO on average occurs approximately 2.5 hours before habitual bedtime.[59] Note that throughout this review, we use the terms *habitual bedtime* and *habitual wake time* as proxies for habitual lights-out and habitual lights-on time. As there is substantial individual variability in the DLMO to bedtime interval,[59] this re-referencing of the PRC from DLMO to habitual bedtime adds in substantial error. Furthermore, as noted previously, there may be significant variability in an individual's sleep schedule, making DLMO predictions based on habitual bedtime even more fraught. Nonetheless, despite all these limitations, there is still useful information to gain from PRCs (**Fig. 4**).

The key principles evident from the PRC to light that are most relevant to light treatment include (1) light in the evening before bedtime and in the first part of habitual sleep phase delays circadian timing, (2) light in the morning from a few hours

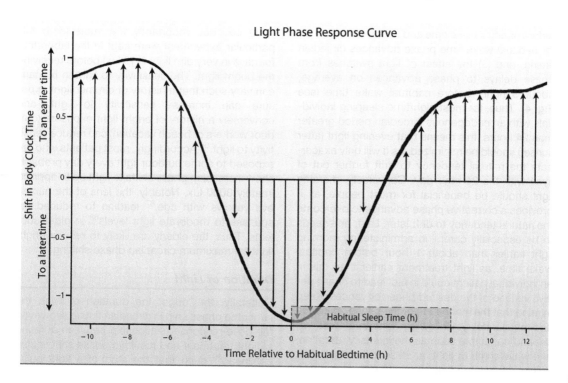

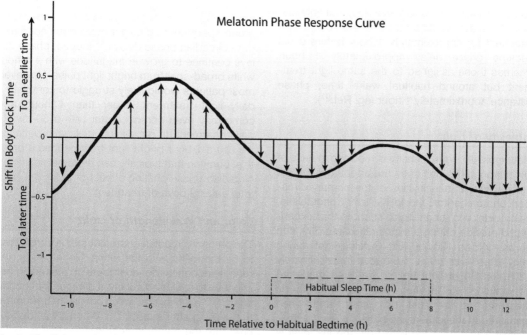

Fig. 4. The light and melatonin phase response curves re-referenced to habitual sleep timing. The light phase response curve is adapted from a phase-response curve generated to a single 1-hour pulse of white broad-spectrum bright light.[55] There is some debate as to whether humans are as sensitive to light during the day as this phase-response curve suggests. The melatonin phase-response curve is adapted from a phase-response curve generated to 3 days of a daily dose of 0.5 mg of exogenous melatonin.[96] Accordingly, we have reduced the amplitude of the melatonin phase-response curve by a factor of 3 to better estimate the effects of a single dose. This phase-response curve may overestimate the phase-shifting effects of exogenous melatonin, as the phase shifts were measured in the absence of a fixed light-dark cycle. As discussed in the main text, phase-response curves are useful general guides, but cannot be used to precisely predict phase shifts in circadian timing in individual patients.

before habitual wake time and for several hours after habitual wake time phase advances circadian timing, and (3) the effect of light switches from phase delays to phase advances on average, about 3 hours before habitual wake time (see **Fig. 4**). Thus, for most nighttime sleeping individuals with an endogenous circadian period greater than 24 hours, this means that evening light (after sunset) should be minimized, as it will only exacerbate the natural tendency to drift further out of sync with the 24-hour day. Conversely, morning light should be beneficial for most people, as it provides a corrective phase advance to overcome the natural tendency to drift later. Last, one needs to be especially careful in administering morning light earlier than about 1 hour before habitual wake time, as light treatment earlier than this in an individual patient could in fact lead to phase delays instead of the desired phase advances. Keep in mind that the magnitude of the phase advances and phase delays following light treatment will depend on factors such as the intensity, duration, and wavelength of light, as described later in this article. Often large individual differences in phase shifts to the same bright light treatment are observed (eg, Ref.[60]). On average, patients assigned to a daily white broad-spectrum bright light treatment for approximately 1 hour before usual bedtime phase delay approximately 1 hour, whereas those assigned to the same light treatment but around habitual wake time, phase advance approximately 1 hour (eg, Ref.[61]).

Intensity of Light

Most typically, light intensity is reported in units of lux, although this unit does not adequately reflect the wavelength sensitivities of the primary circadian photoreceptor, the ipRGCs.[62] Nonetheless, as a guide, very bright light, such as that experienced outside during a sunny cloudless day, can be as high as 100,000 lux. Outside light during rainy days can often be above approximately 1000 lux. Bright light boxes are often marketed as emitting 10,000 lux, but that intensity is measured at the light box itself, and when measured at the level of the patient's eye approximately 2 feet from the light box, the lux level is closer to approximately 3000 to 5000 lux. Indoor light is typically only approximately 100 to 200 lux, although at night people typically experience less than 40 lux in their homes.[63,64]

Light of greater intensity is often associated with larger phase shifts, but importantly, the dose-response relationship is nonlinear.[65] The most detailed dose-response curve suggests maximum phase shifts in humans occur at approximately 1000 lux, but importantly the subjects in this particular experiment were kept in the laboratory for days in very dim light (<10 lux) before receiving the bright light. The sensitivity to light in humans can vary such that a history of dimmer light exposure can increase sensitivity to light, and conversely a history of bright light exposure (outdoor workers or beach vacation) can reduce sensitivity to light.[66] Accordingly, most patients who are exposed to some outdoor light every day probably show increasing phase shifts to light up to approximately 3000 lux. Notably, the lens of the human eye yellows with age,[67] leading to reduced responses to moderate light levels[68] in older subjects. Thus, the elderly are likely to require bright light for maximum circadian phase shifting.

Duration of Light

Generally, the longer the duration of light, the larger the phase shift in circadian timing. However, the dose-response relationship between duration of light treatment and resulting phase shift is also nonlinear,[69] such that the start of a light pulse can often have more of a phase-shifting effect than the rest of the light pulse. The most detailed dose-response curve suggests a 1-hour white broad-spectrum bright light pulse does not maximize circadian phase delays.[69] Indeed, phase delays continue to grow in magnitude with a 4-hour white broad-spectrum bright light pulse. However, most patients would likely struggle to complete a daily light treatment longer than 1 hour, and some may even comply better with a 30-minute daily treatment. In our clinical trials with patients, we use a 1-hour bright light treatment as a practical duration that typically can produce significant circadian phase-shifting effects of at least 1 hour after several days of treatment.

Color and Wavelength of Light

The primary circadian photoreceptor is considered to be the ipRGCs in the retina. Nonetheless, the rods and cones do contribute to circadian responses to light, particularly in dimmer light conditions,[70,71] such as that which occurs in the home in the evening after sunset.[63,64] When it was discovered that the photopigment in the ipRGCs, melanopsin, is maximally sensitive to blue or short wavelength (~480 nm) light,[72,73] researchers and clinicians wondered if larger phase shifts could be generated with blue light. However, to date there is no evidence that monochromatic blue light boxes can lead to greater phase shifts than white broad-spectrum bright light boxes.[74] Similarly, white broad-spectrum bright light boxes with additional blue photons ("blue-enriched") produce similar phase advances and phase delays to white broad-spectrum bright light boxes.[75,76] The lack of an additional phase shift is likely due to the bright light boxes already saturating the retinal receptors, and thus phase shifts cannot be increased. Nonetheless, at dimmer light intensities that do not saturate the retinal receptors, blue light can produce larger phase shifts than white broad-spectrum light.[77]

PRACTICAL ASPECTS OF LIGHT TREATMENT
Light Outdoors

When morning bright light can be found outdoors, patients who need morning light treatment should consider a reorganization of their morning schedule (eg, dog walking, outdoor exercise without sunglasses) to increase their morning light exposure. However, light devices are needed for when circumstances do not allow for this, such as with inclement weather, or when evening or nighttime light treatment is required.

Light Boxes

Light boxes, in a variety of shapes and sizes, come on and off the market at various times. Often the choice of a particular light box will vary according to each individual patient's circumstances and preference. In general, we prefer larger white broad-spectrum bright light boxes, as they generate a larger field of bright light that is easier to stay within, ensuring adequate light exposure. However, these larger light boxes are somewhat cumbersome to move and therefore are best for patients who will receive their light treatment in the same place each day (most typically at home). Smaller light boxes are much more portable and, when battery operated, are particularly easy to take traveling internationally. But it is easier to move out of the range of light exposure emitted from smaller light boxes. As described previously, there is no evidence to date to suggest that blue monochromatic or blue-enriched white broad-spectrum bright light is more effective than white broad-spectrum bright light, but if some patients find the brighter light levels aversive, they may prefer the dimmer devices that emit more blue wavelengths. If a smaller light box is used, it may be useful for patients to periodically check their faces in a mirror to confirm they are receiving sufficient light.[78]

In our laboratory-based studies, we have found a single broad-spectrum bright light box works well to shift circadian timing providing it is set up correctly. **Fig. 5** illustrates the use of such a light box (EnergyLight HF3318/60; Philips, Inc, Andover, MA, USA). A particular advantage

of this model of light box is that it can tip forward toward the patient from its base. We tape a 2-foot-long string to the base of the light box and the patient pulls the string out to his or her eyes during light treatment to ensure the patient is sitting close enough. Note with one light box in front of the patient, the ideal activity during the light treatment is to either read or use an e-tablet, flat on the table in front of the subject so as not to diminish the amount of light reaching the eyes. We also ask patients to turn on their indoor lighting during the light treatment to maximum intensity to optimize the light treatment. Patients should not sleep immediately after a morning light treatment as this "dark pulse" can counteract the effects of the morning light.

In our home-based clinical research trials we find that more than half of the patients wish to either watch TV or use a computer during a daily 1-hour bright light treatment. To ensure adequate bright light still reaches both eyes, we then use 2 light boxes, which are set up to face the patient but are angled slightly to the right and left so that the patient can view the computer screen or TV directly in front of the patient.[79] If the light set up occurs in the living room, side tables are brought in to support the light boxes, and the light set up often creates a considerable change to the layout of the room, potentially interfering with the use of the space by other family members. A better option, when possible, is to set the light boxes up in a room separate from the living space, such as a spare bedroom or study.

Dawn Simulators and Light Masks

There has been some interest in shifting circadian timing with light administration *during* sleep. Commercially available dawn simulators are light boxes designed to be placed near the bed and set to start increasing light in the 30 minutes or so before usual wake time, sometimes remaining on in the first 30 minutes or so after habitual wake time. They are typically not as bright as standard light boxes, reaching lower peak intensities (eg, ~250 lux). Although dawn simulators can improve mood and alertness, the evidence on whether or not they can shift circadian timing is mixed. Some studies report that a single morning exposure, and a 2-week treatment with a dawn simulator did not shift circadian timing.[80,81] However, others report a 3-week treatment produced small phase advances in circadian timing (~30 minutes).[82] As only approximately 1% to 2% of the more potent blue/green light wavelengths passes through closed eyelids,[83] the light from dawn simulators will be most effective when it wakes patients early,

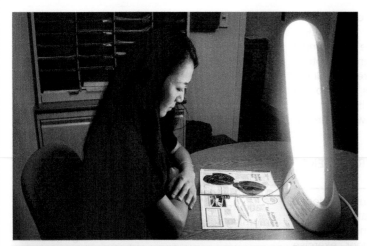

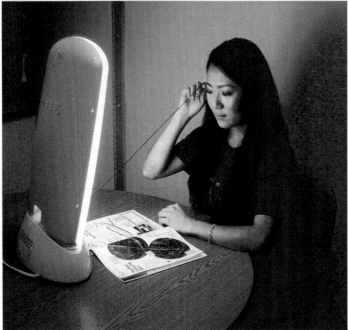

Fig. 5. A member of our research staff demonstrates receiving light treatment from a white broad-spectrum bright light box. A 2-feet-long string attached to the base can remind patients of how close they need to sit to the light box to receive light of greater than 3000 lux.

causing them to open their eyes while the light is on. Currently, there is not enough evidence to conclusively recommend dawn simulators for phase advancing, but they may be an option for patients who are otherwise unlikely to complete a daily morning light treatment.

Light masks, designed to administer light during sleep, have been developed.[84,85] The masks are designed to emit bright light such that light of sufficient intensity still reaches the retina after passing through closed eyelids, without major disruption to sleep. There is preliminary evidence that light masks can shift circadian timing,[84,85] and they appear to be well tolerated. Nonetheless, more testing of light masks is required and to our knowledge no light masks are currently commercially available.

Light Visors and Light Glasses

A significant problem with light boxes is that the patient needs to sit in front of the light box for 30 to 60 minutes per day. One study that examined adherence to a daily light box treatment found that on average patients only self-administer approximately 59% of a prescribed light treatment.[86] An alternative to light boxes are head worn light devices. There is some evidence that light visors, in which the light source is positioned above the eyes, can phase shift circadian timing.[87,88] One type of light glasses, the Re-timer (Re-time, Inc, Adelaide, SA, Australia), has recently become commercially available (**Fig. 6**). In this device, the light source is positioned below the eyes, and there is some evidence that an

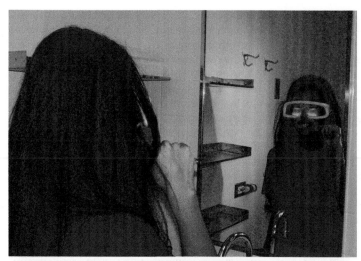

Fig. 6. A member of our research staff demonstrates receiving light treatment from a Re-timer. Patients can freely move around while receiving light treatment, and can complete household activities.

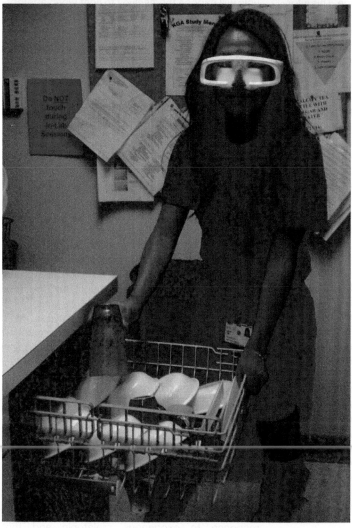

earlier prototype of these glasses could shift circadian timing.[89] Importantly, these head-worn light devices are highly portable, and permit the patient to engage in household activities during their light treatment. Thus, these light devices may improve compliance to light treatment, although this remains to be conclusively demonstrated.

Most light devices do not record their on/off times for later review by clinicians, despite evidence that patients' reports of light treatment can overestimate duration of light treatment.[86] In our home-based clinical trials, we tape a photosensor (Actiwatch Spectrum; Philips, Inc) facing inward on the bottom of the light box, near the stand, to record when the light box is turned on. Ideally, in the future, light devices will record their on and off times, just as, for example, continuous positive airway pressure machines for sleep apnea record their usage. This information will help the clinician understand if a poor treatment response is due to potential minimal use or even use at the wrong time, or if the patient has been compliant to the prescribed light treatment.

Light Avoidance

To facilitate circadian phase shifts to either light treatment and/or exogenous melatonin, light exposure at inappropriate times can be avoided or reduced. For example, night shift workers wishing to phase delay, can wear dark sunglasses during their morning commute home to reduce their exposure to phase advancing morning light.[90] Conversely, patients needing to phase advance, can reduce their evening light exposure with the use of blue blocker orange glasses, which block the blue wavelengths of light the circadian system is most sensitive to.[91] We have found that dimming indoor lights in the evening combined with evening use of blue blockers, phase advanced the DLMO by approximately 1 hour, as compared with maximizing indoor lighting in the evening.[92] On average, subjects wore the blue blockers for approximately 70% of the prescribed 4 hours, but there was considerable individual variability (10%–98%). There is also much interest in reducing exposure to potentially phase delaying light-emitting electronics in the evening, as these devices emit blue wavelength light that the circadian system is most sensitive to.[93] This can be done by dimming the screen, using devices with smaller screens, wearing blue blockers, and overall reducing evening use of electronic devices that are brought close to the eyes, such as e-tablets and cell phones.

Light/Dark Scheduling

As noted previously, it is not uncommon for patients to have irregular sleep/wake schedules that beget variable light/dark patterns. Light treatment and the strategic avoidance of light therefore have the potential to simply add to the existing light/dark variability. For this reason, it is important to ensure that light avoidance and/or light treatments occur at a consistent time from day to day. In our clinical practice, we often recommend the use of alarms, device alerts, and outlet timers (for non–battery-powered electronic devices) to help patients develop a consistent light/dark schedule. Such aids are important for enforcing both regular lights-on and *lights-out* times. In such cases, it is important to make the distinction for the patient between a consistent light/dark schedule, that is, under the patient's control, and a consistent sleep/wake schedule that is often out of the patient's control. Finally, many individuals will expose themselves to light when attempting stimulus control therapy, a mainstay of cognitive-behavioral therapy for insomnia that involves getting out of bed when unable to sleep. This also has the *potential* to cause circadian resetting, especially in dark-adapted individuals.

USING MELATONIN AND OTHER MELATONIN RECEPTOR AGONISTS TO SHIFT CIRCADIAN TIMING

Melatonin (N-Acetyl-5-methoxytryptamine) is a hormone secreted by the pineal gland. In both nocturnal and diurnal (day-active) animals it is secreted during the nighttime and as such can be thought of as a marker for the biological night. As first shown by Redman and colleagues,[94] *exogenous* melatonin administration is capable of resetting the circadian pacemaker to both an earlier and later time (phase advance and phase delay, respectively). Subsequent studies have shown this to be true in humans as well.[27,95,96] There are 2 melatonin receptor subtypes, MT1 and MT2, and there is evidence demonstrating that both help to mediate the circadian resetting effects of melatonin.[97,98]

Timing of Melatonin

Exogenous melatonin, like light, shows differential resetting of the circadian pacemaker based on the biological time of administration and, as with light, this can be represented graphically using a PRC. The same caveats noted previously for light PRCs apply to melatonin PRCs as well. Namely, that PRCs average data across many subjects and may not accurately predict an individual's response to exogenous melatonin and that habitual sleep timing provides only a rough approximation of circadian phase. One additional caveat that applies to the melatonin PRCs is that multiple daily doses were administered over 3 to 4 days in a manner analogous to earlier "3-pulse" light PRCs. With these caveats in mind, several PRCs have been published in humans (eg, Refs.[27,96]) and they generally show (1) phase advances when exogenous melatonin is administered in the late afternoon and evening before habitual bedtime with maximum phase advances generally occurring approximately 5 to 7 hours before habitual bedtime, (2) phase delays when exogenous melatonin is administered in the late night and early morning with maximum phase delays generally occurring a couple of hours after habitual wake time, and (3) the effect of melatonin switches from phase advances to phase delays just before habitual bedtime (see **Fig. 4**). Thus, for most individuals sleeping at conventional times, melatonin administration causes maximal shifts in the biological clock when patients are habitually awake (ie, either in the late afternoon for phase advances or the morning after awakening for phase delays). As discussed later in this article, this can necessitate selection of a dose that does not result in soporific effects. Last, one should be aware that although the administration of exogenous melatonin just before or during the habitual sleep episode would be expected to cause phase delays (see **Fig. 4**), there exists the potential for phase advances during this period of time.[96]

Dose of Melatonin

A variety of exogenous melatonin doses have been examined for circadian resetting.[27,96,99,100] There is evidence of a dose-response relationship at lower doses of 0.02 and 0.30 mg.[100] By contrast, when 0.5 mg and 3.0 mg were compared across a range of administration times, maximum phase advances and phase delays were similar.[96] Even higher doses of exogenous melatonin ($\geq$10 mg) may result in a *smaller* resetting effect.[99,101] This initially counterintuitive finding is likely because increasing the dose of exogenous melatonin simultaneously increases the concentration of melatonin in the circulation and *the duration of administration or exposure*. Initially, increases in dose simply cause increased resetting effects,[100] but as higher doses are used, exogenous melatonin levels remain elevated in the circulation for longer periods of time. As a result, additional parts of the melatonin PRC may be stimulated, resulting in less net circadian resetting (ie, a less discrete time signal is provided). Such "spill over"[101] of melatonin onto the "wrong" portion of the melatonin PRC is possible, despite a half-life of just about an hour, because even 0.5-mg to 1.0-mg doses of melatonin can produce supraphysiological levels over several hours or more.[27,102] Melatonin also has well-demonstrated soporific effects,[102–104] although, at least at 0.3-mg and 5.0-mg doses, this effect was confined to circadian times when endogenous melatonin levels were low (ie, the biological day).[105] Therefore, care should be taken to use the lowest dose possible when exogenous melatonin is taken during the habitual waking hours, as is often necessary for maximal circadian resetting effects.

Formulation and Melatonin Agonists

Recent years have seen the introduction of a variety of approved melatonin receptor agonists and melatonin preparations, all of which are MT1 and MT2 melatonin receptor agonists. These include ramelteon, for the treatment of insomnia; agomelatine, which is also a serotonin 5-HT2c antagonist, approved in Europe and Australia for the treatment of depression; tasimelteon, which was approved by the FDA in 2014 for the treatment of the circadian rhythm sleep disorder non–24-hour sleep-wake disorder (non-24), and Circadin, an extended release formulation of 2.0 mg melatonin approved in Europe and Australia for the treatment of primary insomnia. Of these 4 drugs, only tasimelteon was developed with circadian resetting in mind and it should be noted that it is the first and only drug approved by the FDA for the treatment of a circadian rhythm sleep disorder.[106] Complete PRCs do not exist for any of these melatonin agonists, although logic and the results of resetting trials suggest that the approximate timing of phase advances and phase delays is similar to that of exogenous melatonin.[107,108] However, variability in the magnitude of phase shifts and in the timing of administration for advance and delay shifts might exist. There are no data demonstrating superior efficacy of one formulation over another for circadian resetting, although intuitively, extended release formulations might be expected to be *less* effective due to the "spillover" effects discussed previously.

PRACTICAL ASPECTS OF MELATONIN AND OTHER MELATONIN AGONIST TREATMENT
Melatonin Preparations

Exogenous melatonin has been classified by the FDA as a dietary supplement, and as such is not subject to the regulation given to pharmaceuticals; the purity and accuracy of dose of exogenous melatonin formulations are not always carefully controlled.[109] There has been recent progress in this area, and the purity and accuracy of doses may improve, particularly those from large well-established supplement manufacturers.[110] Meanwhile, choosing an over-the-counter formulation from a manufacturer who participates in the US Pharmacopeia Verified Program for Dietary Supplements may help with this quality control problem.[111] Consumers can also pay to access the results of consumer group testing of various melatonin brands and formulations.[112] An important consideration for therapy with melatonin is the low cost (often <10 cents per pill[112]).

Issues of dose are discussed in more detail earlier in this article, but the clinician should be aware that commonly available doses (0.5 mg and 3.0 mg) demonstrate equivalent resetting effects,[96] whereas evidence of diminished efficacy with higher doses ("spill over") appears at doses of 10 mg and higher. With this in mind, the clinician should choose the lowest dose with demonstrated efficacy and lower it further if unwanted sedation occurs. Caution should be exercised with the first dose, as with a sedative-hypnotic, to ensure that excessive sedation does not occur. Finally, pharmacokinetic data show that even doses as low as 0.5 to 1.0 mg may result in supra-physiologic levels of melatonin.[27,102]

Melatonin Administration

As with light administration, the clinician should ideally help the patient to adopt as consistent of a light/dark schedule as possible first. This may be therapeutic in its own right, and it also allows for a better prediction of circadian phase based on habitual sleep times. It is important to make sure that melatonin is not in competition with either the self-selected light/dark cycle or light therapy. It should be noted that the most current melatonin PRC was constructed in the laboratory without competing light resetting[96] and, as might be expected, it showed somewhat greater phase shifts than a PRC based on melatonin administered while subjects lived at home.[27] If symptoms are improved but the timing of sleep remains delayed or advanced, the timing of administration can be slowly advanced or delayed an hour,[113] or less, every several days, as tolerated by the patient, in concert with the timing of light and dark such that the relationship to habitual sleep/wake and light/dark times is maintained. Patients can be reminded to take melatonin with the use of alarms of various sorts, including setting a daily alarm on their cell phones.

A special case exists for the treatment of the circadian rhythm sleep disorder non-24 in which circadian phase drifts progressively later, and sometimes earlier, each day due to a lack of synchronization of the biological clock (typically due to a loss of photic input in totally blind individuals). The clinician must be especially mindful of timing the administration of melatonin or melatonin agonist in such a way as to promote a normal relationship between the timing of the clock and the desired timing of sleep (ie, a DLMO ~2–3 hours before bedtime). Studies have shown that the final entrained DLMO can occur roughly 0 to 5 hours *after* the time of administration depending on the dose.[100,114] Therefore, administration 3 to 8 hours before desired bedtime may be necessary. We recommend an initial administration time of 6 hours before the desired bedtime. If the patient shows evidence of being phase advanced, the time of administration can be delayed to a later time (and vice versa). A small minority of blind individuals drift to a progressively earlier time.[25] In these cases, administration of melatonin just after the desired wake time has been shown to appropriately set the biological clock relative to sleep.[115]

Finally, potential interactions with other prescription medications and/or other over-the-counter dietary supplements should be considered (see potential contraindications listed earlier in this article). Unfortunately, there are indications that fewer than half of the general population does so.[3]

Melatonin and Light Combination Treatment

It has been shown that afternoon melatonin can increase the phase advances obtained with morning light administration.[116–118] It has yet to be shown that phase delays obtained with evening light treatment can be increased with morning melatonin. To our knowledge, there have been no studies to date on light treatment in combination with other melatonin receptor agonists.

EVALUATION OF OUTCOME

In practice, treatment response is largely assessed on the basis of symptom improvement in circadian rhythm sleep disorders, as there are currently no FDA-approved laboratory assessments of circadian phase (ie, no current clinical DLMO test). Subjective sleep diary or, if available, more objective wrist actigraphy measures of sleep timing and relevant sleep variables, such as sleep-onset latency, total sleep time, and early morning awakening, are useful. In the case of non-24 in the blind, spectral analysis of wrist actigraphy data has the potential to be a cost-effective method of assessing entrainment status and therefore treatment efficacy.[25] Similar to oral contraceptives, consistent timing in light and/or exogenous melatonin treatment is important for efficacy and this should be assessed as well (eg, by diary or medication compliance bottles) before determinations of efficacy are made.

SUMMARY

There is increasing recognition of the important influence circadian timing has on mental health, physical health, and health behaviors. In this review, we provided a brief summary of the circadian system, followed by some of the initial considerations to make when considering treating a patient with suspected circadian misalignment. A consistent light/dark schedule should first be attempted, followed by a consideration of contradictions and safety concerns associated with light and exogenous melatonin treatment. If the patient has no contraindications for light treatment, decisions regarding the timing, intensity, duration, color of light, and the possibility for complementary light avoidance need to be made. Patient input, particularly their motivation to engage in an often-required daily treatment, should guide the choice of light device. If the patient has no contraindications for exogenous melatonin treatment, decisions regarding the timing, dose, slow-release or fast-release formulation, purity, and the possible use of other melatonin receptor agonists needs to be made. Currently, treatment response is largely assessed based on symptom improvement.

ACKNOWLEDGMENTS

We thank Muneer Rizvydeen for his assistance in creating the figures. We thank Haein Sung for allowing us to include photos of her during light treatment. H.J. Burgess is supported by grants from the National Center for Complementary and Integrative Health (AT007104), and the National Institute on Alcohol Abuse and Alcoholism (AA021762). The content is solely the responsibility of the authors and does not necessarily represent the official views of the National Institutes of Health.

REFERENCES

1. Lam RW, Levitt AJ. Canadian consensus guidelines for the treatment of seasonal affective disorder. (Canada): Clinical & Academic Publishing; 1999. p. 160.
2. National Sleep Foundation. Sleep in America poll. 2005. Available at: www.sleepfoundation.org. Accessed July 21, 2015.
3. Bliwise DL, Ansari FP. Insomnia associated with valerian and melatonin usage in the 2002 National Health Interview Survey. Sleep 2007;30:881–4.
4. Wright KP Jr, Hull JT, Hughes RJ, et al. Sleep and wakefulness out of phase with internal biological time impairs learning in humans. J Cogn Neurosci 2006;18:508–21.
5. Scheer FA, Hilton MF, Mantzoros CS, et al. Adverse metabolic and cardiovascular consequences of circadian misalignment. Proc Natl Acad Sci U S A 2009;106:4453–8.
6. Levandovski R, Dantas G, Fernandes LC, et al. Depression scores associate with chronotype and social jetlag in a rural population. Chronobiol Int 2011;28:771–8.
7. Bartness TJ, Song CK, Demas GE. SCN efferents to peripheral tissues: implications for biological rhythms. J Biol Rhythms 2001;16:196–204.
8. Buijs RM, Scheer FA, Kreier F, et al. Organization of circadian functions: interaction with the body. Prog Brain Res 2006;153:341–60.
9. Dijk DJ, von Schantz M. Timing and consolidation of human sleep, wakefulness, and performance by a symphony of oscillators. J Biol Rhythms 2005;20:279–90.
10. Scheiermann C, Kunisaki Y, Lucas D, et al. Adrenergic nerves govern circadian leukocyte recruitment to tissues. Immunity 2012;37:290–301.
11. Buhr ED, Yoo SH, Takahashi JS. Temperature as a universal resetting cue for mammalian circadian oscillators. Science 2010;330:379–85.
12. Lewy AJ, Wehr TA, Goodwin FK, et al. Light suppresses melatonin secretion in humans. Science 1980;210:1267–9.
13. Gaggioni G, Maquet P, Schmidt C, et al. Neuroimaging, cognition, light and circadian rhythms. Front Syst Neurosci 2014;8:126.
14. DeMuro RL, Nafziger AN, Blask DE, et al. The absolute bioavailability of oral melatonin. J Clin Pharmacol 2000;40:781–4.
15. Auger RR, Burgess HJ, Emens JS, et al. Clinical practice guideline for the treatment of intrinsic circadian rhythm sleep-wake disorders: advanced sleep-wake phase disorder (ASWPD), delayed sleep-wake phase disorder (DSWPD), non-24-hour sleepwake rhythm disorder (N24SWD), and irregular sleep-wake rhythm disorder (ISWRD). J Clin Sleep Med 2015, in press.
16. Guaiana G, Gupta S, Chiodo D, et al. Agomelatine versus other antidepressive agents for major depression. Cochrane Database Syst Rev 2013;(12):CD008851.
17. Lewy AJ, Lefler BJ, Emens JS, et al. The circadian basis of winter depression. Proc Natl Acad Sci U S A 2006;103:7414–9.
18. Neubauer DN. New and emerging pharmacotherapeutic approaches for insomnia. Int Rev Psychiatry 2014;26:214–24.
19. Lucas RJ, Lall GS, Allen AE, et al. How rod, cone, and melanopsin photoreceptors come together to

enlighten the mammalian circadian clock. Prog Brain Res 2012;199:1–18.

20. Reppert SM, Weaver DR, Rivkees SA, et al. Putative melatonin receptors in a human biological clock. Science 1988;242:78–81.

21. Moore RY. Organization and function of a central nervous system circadian oscillator: the suprachiasmatic nucleus. Fed Proc 1983;42:2783–9.

22. Burgess HJ, Eastman CI. Human tau in an ultradian light-dark cycle. J Biol Rhythms 2008;23:374–6.

23. Duffy JF, Cain SW, Chang AM, et al. Sex difference in the near-24-hour intrinsic period of the human circadian timing system. Proc Natl Acad Sci U S A 2011;108(Suppl 3):15602–8.

24. National Sleep Foundation. Sleep in America poll. 2011. Available at: www.sleepfoundation.org. Accessed July 21, 2015.

25. Emens JS, Laurie AL, Songer JB, et al. Non-24-hour disorder in blind individuals revisited: variability and the influence of environmental time cues. Sleep 2013;36:1091–100.

26. Moore RY. Neural control of the pineal gland. Behav Brain Res 1996;73:125–30.

27. Lewy AJ, Bauer VK, Ahmed S, et al. The human phase response curve (PRC) to melatonin is about 12 hours out of phase with the PRC to light. Chronobiol Int 1998;15:71–83.

28. Klerman EB, Gershengorn HB, Duffy JF, et al. Comparisons of the variability of three markers of the human circadian pacemaker. J Biol Rhythms 2002;17:181–93.

29. Lewy AJ, Cutler NL, Sack RL. The endogenous melatonin profile as a marker of circadian phase position. J Biol Rhythms 1999;14:227–36.

30. Benloucif S, Burgess HJ, Klerman EB, et al. Measuring melatonin in humans. J Clin Sleep Med 2008;4:66–9.

31. Molina TA, Burgess HJ. Calculating the dim light melatonin onset: the impact of threshold and sampling rate. Chronobiol Int 2011;28:714–8.

32. Nicolaides NC, Charmandari E, Chrousos GP, et al. Circadian endocrine rhythms: the hypothalamic-pituitary-adrenal axis and its actions. Ann N Y Acad Sci 2014;1318:71–80.

33. Challet E. Circadian clocks, food intake, and metabolism. Prog Mol Biol Transl Sci 2013;119:105–35.

34. Emens J, Lewy A, Kinzie JM, et al. Circadian misalignment in major depressive disorder. Psychiatry Res 2009;168:259–61.

35. Boivin DB. Influence of sleep-wake and circadian rhythm disturbances in psychiatric disorders. J Psychiatry Neurosci 2000;25:446–58.

36. Roenneberg T, Wirz-Justice A, Merrow M. Life between clocks: daily temporal patterns of human chronotypes. J Biol Rhythms 2003;18:80–90.

37. Wittmann M, Dinich J, Merrow M, et al. Social jet-lag: misalignment of biological and social time. Chronobiol Int 2006;23:497–509.

38. Kanerva N, Kronholm E, Partonen T, et al. Tendency toward eveningness is associated with unhealthy dietary habits. Chronobiol Int 2012;29:920–7.

39. Van den Hoofdakker RH. Chronobiological theories of nonseasonal affective disorders and their implications for treatment. J Biol Rhythms 1994;9:157–83.

40. Pail G, Huf W, Pjrek E, et al. Bright-light therapy in the treatment of mood disorders. Neuropsychobiology 2011;64:152–62.

41. Terman M, Terman JS. Light therapy for seasonal and nonseasonal depression: efficacy, protocol, safety, and side effects. CNS Spectr 2005;10:647–63.

42. Gallin PF, Terman M, Reme CE, et al. Ophthalmologic examination of patients with seasonal affective disorder, before and after bright light therapy. Am J Ophthalmol 1995;119:202–10.

43. Herxheimer A, Petrie KJ. Melatonin for the prevention and treatment of jet lag. Cochrane Database Syst Rev 2002;(2):CD001520.

44. Buscemi N, Vandermeer B, Hooton N, et al. The efficacy and safety of exogenous melatonin for primary sleep disorders. A meta-analysis. J Gen Intern Med 2005;20:1151–8.

45. Valcavi R, Zini M, Maestroni GJ, et al. Melatonin stimulates growth hormone secretion through pathways other than the growth hormone-releasing hormone. Clin Endocrinol (Oxf) 1993;39:193–9.

46. van Geijlswijk IM, Mol RH, Egberts TC, et al. Evaluation of sleep, puberty and mental health in children with long-term melatonin treatment for chronic idiopathic childhood sleep onset insomnia. Psychopharmacology (Berl) 2010;216:111–20.

47. McMullan CJ, Schernhammer ES, Rimm EB, et al. Melatonin secretion and the incidence of type 2 diabetes. JAMA 2013;309:1388–96.

48. Rubio-Sastre P, Scheer FA, Gomez-Abellan P, et al. Acute melatonin administration in humans impairs glucose tolerance in both the morning and evening. Sleep 2014;37:1715–9.

49. Freiesleben SD, Furczyk K. A systematic review of agomelatine-induced liver injury. J Mol Psychiatry 2015;3:4.

50. Taylor D, Sparshatt A, Varma S, et al. Antidepressant efficacy of agomelatine: meta-analysis of published and unpublished studies. BMJ 2014;348:g1888.

51. Available at: http://www.fda.gov/downloads/Advisory-Committees/CommitteesMeetingMaterials/Drugs/PeripheralandCentralNervousSystemDrugsAdvisory-Committee/UCM374385.pdf. Accessed July 21, 2015.

52. Kuriyama A, Honda M, Hayashino Y. Ramelteon for the treatment of insomnia in adults: a systematic review and meta-analysis. Sleep Med 2014;15: 385–92.

53. Available at: http://www.ema.europa.eu/docs/en_GB/document_library/EPAR_-_Summary_for_the_public/human/000695/WC500026805.pdf. Accessed July 21, 2015.

54. Sheldon SH. Pro-convulsant effects of oral melatonin in neurologically disabled children. Lancet 1998;351:1254.

55. St Hilaire MA, Gooley JJ, Khalsa SB, et al. Human phase response curve to a 1h pulse of bright white light. J Physiol 2012;590:3035–45.

56. Dumont M, Carrier J. Daytime sleep propensity after moderate circadian phase shifts induced with bright light exposure. Sleep 1997;20:11–7.

57. Buxton OM, L'Hermite-Baleriaux M, Turek FW, et al. Daytime naps in darkness phase shift the human circadian rhythms of melatonin and thyrotropin secretion. Am J Physiol Regul Integr Comp Physiol 2000;278:R373–82.

58. Burgess HJ, Wyatt JK, Park M, et al. Home circadian phase assessments with measures of compliance yield accurate dim light melatonin onsets. Sleep 2015;38:889–97.

59. Burgess HJ, Fogg LF. Individual differences in the amount and timing of salivary melatonin secretion. PLoS One 2008;3:e3055.

60. Burgess HJ. Partial sleep deprivation reduces phase advances to light in humans. J Biol Rhythms 2010;25:460–8.

61. Burgess HJ, Fogg LF, Young MA, et al. Bright light therapy for winter depression—is phase advancing beneficial? Chronobiol Int 2004;21:759–75.

62. Lucas RJ, Peirson SN, Berson DM, et al. Measuring and using light in the melanopsin age. Trends Neurosci 2014;37:1–9.

63. Burgess HJ, Eastman CI. Early versus late bedtimes phase shift the human dim light melatonin rhythm despite a fixed morning lights on time. Neurosci Lett 2004;356:115–8.

64. Crowley SJ, Molina TA, Burgess HJ. A week in the life of full-time office workers: work day and weekend light exposure in summer and winter. Appl Ergon 2015;46 Pt A:193–200.

65. Zeitzer JM, Dijk DJ, Kronauer RE, et al. Sensitivity of the human circadian pacemaker to nocturnal light: melatonin phase resetting and suppression. J Physiol 2000;526 Pt 3:695–702.

66. Hebert M, Martin SK, Lee C, et al. The effects of prior light history on the suppression of melatonin by light in humans. J Pineal Res 2002;33:198–203.

67. Weale RA. Age and the transmittance of the human crystalline lens. J Physiol 1988;395:577–87.

68. Duffy JF, Zeitzer JM, Czeisler CA. Decreased sensitivity to phase-delaying effects of moderate intensity light in older subjects. Neurobiol Aging 2007;28:799–807.

69. Chang AM, Santhi N, St Hilaire MA, et al. Human responses to bright light of different durations. J Physiol 2012;590:3103–12.

70. Lall GS, Revell VL, Momiji H, et al. Distinct contributions of rod, cone and melanopsin photoreceptors to encoding irradiance. Neuron 2010;66:417–28.

71. Walmsley L, Hanna L, Mouland J, et al. Colour as a signal for entraining the mammalian circadian clock. PLoS Biol 2015;13:e1002127.

72. Thapan K, Arendt J, Skene DJ. An action spectrum for melatonin suppression: evidence for a novel non-rod, non-cone photoreceptor system in humans. J Physiol 2001;535:261–7.

73. Brainard GC, Hanifin JP, Greeson JM, et al. Action spectrum for melatonin regulation in humans: evidence for a novel circadian photoreceptor. J Neurosci 2001;21:6405–12.

74. Revell VL, Molina TA, Eastman CI. Human phase response curve to intermittent blue light using a commercially available device. J Physiol 2012; 590:4859–68.

75. Smith MR, Eastman CI. Phase delaying the human circadian clock with blue-enriched polychromatic light. Chronobiol Int 2009;26:709–25.

76. Smith MR, Revell VL, Eastman CI. Phase advancing the human circadian clock with blue-enriched polychromatic light. Sleep Med 2009;10: 287–94.

77. Mottram V, Middleton B, Williams P, et al. The impact of bright artificial white and 'blue-enriched' light on sleep and circadian phase during the polar winter. J Sleep Res 2011;20:154–61.

78. Crowley SJ, Carskadon MA. Modifications to weekend recovery sleep delay circadian phase in older adolescents. Chronobiol Int 2010;27:1469–92.

79. Campbell SS, Dawson D, Anderson MW. Alleviation of sleep maintenance insomnia with timed exposure to bright light. J Am Geriatr Soc 1993;41:829–36.

80. Gabel V, Maire M, Reichert CF, et al. Effects of artificial dawn and morning blue light on daytime cognitive performance, well-being, cortisol and melatonin levels. Chronobiol Int 2013;30:988–97.

81. Gimenez MC, Hessels M, van de Werken M, et al. Effects of artificial dawn on subjective ratings of sleep inertia and dim light melatonin onset. Chronobiol Int 2010;27:1219–41.

82. Terman M, Terman JS. Circadian rhythm phase advance with dawn simulation treatment for winter depression. J Biol Rhythms 2010;25:297–301.

83. Moseley MJ, Bayliss SC, Fielder AR. Light transmission through the human eyelid: in vivo measurement. Ophthalmic Physiol Opt 1988;8:229–30.

84. Cole RJ, Smith JS, Alcala YC, et al. Bright-light mask treatment of delayed sleep phase syndrome. J Biol Rhythms 2002;17:89–101.

85. Figueiro MG, Rea MS. Preliminary evidence that light through the eyelids can suppress melatonin and phase shift dim light melatonin onset. BMC Res Notes 2012;5:221.

86. Michalak EE, Murray G, Wilkinson C, et al. A pilot study of adherence with light treatment for seasonal affective disorder. Psychiatry Res 2007;149: 315–20.

87. Boulos Z, Macchi MM, Sturchler MP, et al. Light visor treatment for jet lag after westward travel across six time zones. Aviat Space Environ Med 2002;73:953–63.

88. Paul MA, Miller JC, Gray G, et al. Circadian phase delay induced by phototherapeutic devices. Aviat Space Environ Med 2007;78:645–52.

89. Wright HR, Lack LC, Partridge KJ. Light emitting diodes can be used to phase delay the melatonin rhythm. J Pineal Res 2001;31:350–5.

90. Burgess HJ, Sharkey KM, Eastman CI. Bright light, dark and melatonin can promote circadian adaptation in night shift workers. Sleep Med Rev 2002;6: 407–20.

91. Sasseville A, Paquet N, Sevigny J, et al. Blue blocker glasses impede the capacity of bright light to suppress melatonin production. J Pineal Res 2006;41:73–8.

92. Burgess HJ, Molina TA. Home lighting before usual bedtime impacts circadian timing: a field study. Photochem Photobiol 2014;90:723–6.

93. Chang AM, Aeschbach D, Duffy JF, et al. Evening use of light-emitting eReaders negatively affects sleep, circadian timing, and next-morning alertness. Proc Natl Acad Sci U S A 2015;112:1232–7.

94. Redman J, Armstrong S, Ng KT. Free-running activity rhythms in the rat: entrainment by melatonin. Science 1983;219:1089–91.

95. Arendt J, Bojkowski C, Folkard S, et al. Some effects of melatonin and the control of its secretion in humans. In: Evered D, Clark S, editors. Photoperiodism, melatonin, and the pineal. London: Pitman; 1985. p. 266–83.

96. Burgess HJ, Revell VL, Molina TA, et al. Human phase response curves to three days of daily melatonin: 0.5 mg versus 3.0 mg. J Clin Endocrinol Metab 2010;95:3325–31.

97. Reppert SM, Weaver DR, Godson C. Melatonin receptors step into the light: cloning and classification of subtypes. Trends Pharmacol Sci 1996;17:100–2.

98. Dubocovich ML. Melatonin receptors: role on sleep and circadian rhythm regulation. Sleep Med 2007; 8(Suppl 3):34–42.

99. Sack RL, Brandes RW, Kendall AR, et al. Entrainment of free-running circadian rhythms by melatonin in blind people. N Engl J Med 2000;343:1070–7.

100. Lewy AJ, Emens JS, Lefler BJ, et al. Melatonin entrains free-running blind people according to a physiological dose-response curve. Chronobiol Int 2005;22:1093–106.

101. Lewy AJ, Emens JS, Sack RL, et al. Low, but not high, doses of melatonin entrained a free-running blind person with long circadian period. Chronobiol Int 2002;19:649–58.

102. Dollins AB, Zhdanova IV, Wurtman RJ, et al. Effect of inducing nocturnal serum melatonin concentrations in daytime on sleep, mood, body temperature, and performance. Proc Natl Acad Sci U S A 1994;91:1824–8.

103. James SP, Mendelson WB, Sack DA, et al. The effect of melatonin on normal sleep. Neuropsychopharmacology 1987;1:41–4.

104. Rajaratnam SMW, Middleton B, Stone BM, et al. Melatonin advances the circadian timing of EEG sleep and directly facilitates sleep without altering its duration in extended sleep opportunities in humans. J Physiol 2004;561:339–51.

105. Wyatt JK, Dijk DJ, Ritz-de Cecco A, et al. Sleep-facilitating effect of exogenous melatonin in healthy young men and women is circadian-phase dependent. Sleep 2006;29:609–18.

106. Available at: http://www.fda.gov/NewsEvents/Newsroom/PressAnnouncements/ucm384092.htm. Accessed July 21, 2015.

107. Rajaratnam SM, Polymeropoulos MH, Fisher DM, et al. Melatonin agonist tasimelteon (VEC-162) for transient insomnia after sleep-time shift: two randomised controlled multicentre trials. Lancet 2009; 373:482–91.

108. Richardson GS, Zee PC, Wang-Weigand S, et al. Circadian phase-shifting effects of repeated ramelteon administration in healthy adults. J Clin Sleep Med 2008;4:456–61.

109. Hahm H, Kujawa J, Augsburger L. Comparison of melatonin products against USP's nutritional supplements standards and other criteria. J Am Pharm Assoc (Wash) 1999;39:27–31.

110. Available at: http://well.blogs.nytimes.com/2015/03/30/gnc-to-strengthen-supplement-quality-controls/?_r=0. Accessed July 21, 2015.

111. Available at: http://www.usp.org/usp-verification-services/usp-verified-dietary-supplements/participating-companies. Accessed July 21, 2015.

112. ConsumerLab.com, product review: melatonin supplements. Available at: www.consumerlab.com/results/melatonin.asp. Accessed August 13, 2012.

113. Crowley SJ, Eastman CI. Melatonin in the afternoons of a gradually advancing sleep schedule enhances the circadian rhythm phase advance. Psychopharmacology (Berl) 2013;225:825–37.

114. Lewy AJ, Emens JS, Bernert RA, et al. Eventual entrainment of the human circadian pacemaker by melatonin is independent of the circadian phase of treatment initiation: clinical implications. J Biol Rhythms 2004;19:68–75.

115. Emens J, Lewy A, Yuhas K, et al. Melatonin entrains free-running blind individuals with circadian periods less than 24 hours. Sleep 2006; 29:A62.

116. Revell VL, Burgess HJ, Gazda CJ, et al. Advancing human circadian rhythms with afternoon melatonin and morning intermittent bright light. J Clin Endocrinol Metab 2006;91:54–9.

117. Paul MA, Gray GW, Lieberman HR, et al. Phase advance with separate and combined melatonin and light treatment. Psychopharmacology (Berl) 2011;214:515–23.

118. Burke TM, Markwald RR, Chinoy ED, et al. Combination of light and melatonin time cues for phase advancing the human circadian clock. Sleep 2013;36:1617–24.

Consequences of Circadian Disruption on Cardiometabolic Health

 CrossMark

Sirimon Reutrakul, MD[a], Kristen L. Knutson, PhD[b],*

KEYWORDS

- Circadian rhythms • Diabetes • Cardiovascular disease • Shift work

KEY POINTS

- Circadian disruption can occur when sleep and/or meal timing occurs out of synchrony with the light-dark cycle (environment) or the central circadian clock (endogenous).
- Circadian disruption is associated with increased risk of impaired cardiometabolic function and associated diseases, including obesity, diabetes, and cardiovascular disease.
- Shift work is associated with severe circadian disruption but even milder delays in bedtime or meals are associated with impaired cardiometabolic function.
- Sleep, meal timing, and light at night could link late chronotype and shift work to circadian disruption.

INTRODUCTION

Cardiovascular disease (CVD), diabetes, and obesity affect millions of people worldwide and the rates of these cardiometabolic diseases are on the rise.[1,2] Cardiometabolic diseases are associated with reduced quality of life, lower life expectancy, and increased economic burden on both the individual and on society.[3–6] Therefore, thorough understanding of all the risk factors for these diseases could contribute to improvement in global health. This article discusses a potentially novel risk factor for cardiometabolic disease: circadian disruption.

Circadian disruption occurs when the endogenous circadian (~24-hour) rhythms are not in synchrony with either the environment or each other. This desynchrony can occur when behaviors such as wake, sleep, and meals are not at an appropriate time relative to the timing of the central circadian clock, which is located in the

hypothalamus, and/or relative the external environment, particularly the light-dark cycle. This article reviews studies that examined cardiometabolic health of shift work, which typically leads to circadian disruption; studies that experimentally disrupted circadian rhythms to determine the effects on cardiometabolic function; and observational studies that examined sleep timing and behavioral chronotype. A few potential mediators linking the chronotype and shift work to circadian disruption and cardiometabolic health are briefly discussed.

OBSERVATIONAL STUDIES OF SHIFT WORK

Shift work does not have a universal definition but can refer to work shifts that occur always at night (permanent night shift) or rotate between different shifts (day, afternoon, night) across the month. Some studies also include work shifts that are simply outside the standard 9:00 AM to 5:00 PM on

Disclosure Statement: S. Reutrakul receives speaker honoraria from Sanofi Aventis and research support from Merck (0000-349). K.L. Knutson is the National Sleep Foundation Poll Fellow.
[a] Division of Endocrinology and Metabolism, Faculty of Medicine Ramathibodi Hospital, Mahidol University, 270 Rama VI Road, Bangkok 10400, Thailand; [b] Section of Pulmonary and Critical Care, Department of Medicine, University of Chicago, 5841 South Maryland Avenue, MC 6076, Chicago, IL 60637, USA
* Corresponding author.
E-mail address: kknutson@medicine.bsd.uchicago.edu

Sleep Med Clin 10 (2015) 455–468
http://dx.doi.org/10.1016/j.jsmc.2015.07.005
1556-407X/15/$ – see front matter © 2015 Elsevier Inc. All rights reserved.

Monday through Friday. Any work shift that requires an individual to be awake at a time that their central circadian clock associates with sleep has the potential to disrupt that individual's circadian rhythms.

Shift work has been associated with an increased risk of numerous cardiometabolic diseases and their risk factors. Several studies have reported that the risk of developing CVD is higher in shift workers compared with day workers.[7–9] Shift workers also often have higher blood pressure or rates of hypertension than day workers.[10–12] One study found that endothelial function, a marker of CVD risk, was reduced in shift workers.[13] Another study reported abnormalities on the electrocardiogram in the shift workers.[14] Shift workers are also reported to have a higher prevalence or incidence of type 2 diabetes.[15] The longer the history of working as a shift worker resulted in greater the risk of developing diabetes.[16] Another study suggested that the risk of diabetes was mediated by body weight.[17] A meta-analyses of 12 studies with 226,652 total participants, including 14,595 diabetes subjects, found that having ever worked shift work was associated with increased prevalence of diabetes (pooled odds ratio [OR] 1.09, 95% confidence interval [CI] 1.05–1.12).[18] This meta-analyses also found significant sex differences in that the association was stronger in men (OR = 1.37, 95% CI 1.20–1.56) than in women (OR = 1.09, 95% CI 1.04–1.14).

There are several risk factors for CVD, including being overweight or obese, dyslipidemia, insulin resistance, and impaired beta cell function in the pancreas. Individuals performing shift work often have larger body mass indices (BMIs) or waist circumferences than those only working on day shifts.[12,19–24] Several studies have found that shift workers have higher levels of either total cholesterol or triglycerides, or lower levels of high-density lipoprotein (HDL) cholesterol.[12,22,25–29] Other studies have reported alterations in markers of glucose metabolism, including hyperglycemia.[29] One study observed worse estimated beta cell function but no differences in estimated insulin resistance in shift workers compared with day workers.[30] Finally, shift workers are also more likely to have the metabolic syndrome, which is a cluster of metabolic abnormalities that increase the risk of CVD and diabetes, including abdominal obesity, insulin resistance, high blood pressure, and dyslipidemia.[31–33]

It is important to acknowledge that not all studies have reported significant differences between shift workers and day workers on some cardiometabolic measures or all subgroups studied.[14,28,34–37] Differences in results could be due to varying effects of age, sex, definition of shift work, or the duration of shift work.

EXPERIMENTAL CIRCADIAN DISRUPTION

Several studies have experimentally manipulated circadian rhythms in healthy volunteers to determine the effect of circadian disruption on cardiometabolic functions (**Table 1** summarizes these studies). In one study, 10 participants underwent a 10-day forced desynchrony protocol in which they slept and consumed isocaloric meals during a recurring cycle of a 28-hour day.[38] Blood samples were taken hourly to measure levels of leptin, insulin, glucose, and cortisol, and blood pressure was measured 4 times while awake. When participants ate and slept 12 hours off from their habitual times, the maximal circadian misalignment, glucose levels increased by 6%. This was mostly due to postprandial, rather than fasting, levels and the glucose levels were in a pre-diabetic range in 3 of 8 participants. This increase in glucose occurred despite a 22% increase in insulin levels, suggesting decreased insulin sensitivity with insufficient beta cell compensation. In addition, the circadian rhythm of cortisol was reversed during circadian misalignment with higher levels at the end of a wake episode and at the beginning of a sleep episode, which could also contribute to hyperglycemia. Circadian misalignment was also associated with a 3% increase in mean arterial pressure during wakefulness. Finally, leptin is a satiety signal involved in appetite regulation and the levels of leptin decreased by 17% after circadian disruption. This study demonstrated numerous changes in markers of cardiometabolic function and could explain some of the observed differences between shift workers and day workers.

A second experimental study of circadian disruption also used the 28-hour day forced desynchrony protocol but with concurrent sleep restriction (5.6 hours/24 hours) for 3 weeks to explore the combined effects of sleep restriction and circadian disruption as commonly experienced by shift workers, followed by 9-day recovery period.[39] They enrolled 21 participants; 11 were younger (mean age 23) and 10 were older (mean age 60). Circadian disruption combined with sleep restriction was associated with an 8% increase in fasting glucose levels and a 14% increase in postprandial glucose levels in response to a standardized breakfast. There was an inadequate pancreatic beta cell response because fasting and postprandial peak insulin levels were significantly reduced (by 12% and 27%, respectively). Circadian disruption combined with sleep restriction also decreased the resting metabolic rate by 8%. The 24-hour levels of leptin were slightly lower after circadian disruption combined with sleep restriction, and ghrelin, which is an orexigenic hormone involved in appetite regulation, were slightly higher. These metabolic changes did not differ significantly between the older and younger participants. These results suggest additional details on potential underlying mechanisms of increased diabetes and obesity risk in shift workers.

A third experimental study was designed to determine whether circadian disruption impairs cardiometabolic function independently from the effects of sleep loss using a parallel group design.[40] One group was allowed 5 hours in bed for 8 days with bedtimes always centered at 03:00 hour (circadian aligned) and the second group had 5 hours in bed but on 4 days the bedtimes were delayed by 8.5 hours (circadian misaligned). Both the circadian aligned and misaligned groups had significantly reduced insulin sensitivity without compensatory insulin response. Furthermore, in the men, the decrease in insulin sensitivity was twice as large when circadian misaligned compared with the circadian-aligned group (there were too few women to examine separately). High-sensitivity C-reactive protein (hs-CRP), which is a marker of inflammation, increased in both groups but increased substantially more in the circadian misaligned group ($+146 \pm 103\%$ vs $+64 \pm 63\%$, $P = .049$). The results of this experimental study support an independent effect of circadian disruption on glucose metabolism and cardiometabolic risk.

Eating at a circadian-inappropriate time (ie, at night) in humans is commonly seen in shift workers and may play a role in the obesity risk. One study simulated shift work to examine the effects on energy metabolism using a whole-room calorimeter.[41] This 6-day inpatient study simulated shift work in 14 adults by having 2 daytime shifts with 8-hour nocturnal sleep opportunity followed by the first night shift, which only allowed a brief 2-hour sleep opportunity, and then 2 additional night shifts with 8-hour sleep opportunities during the day. Compared with baseline, total daily energy expenditure was 4% higher on the first night shift but 3% lower on the 2 subsequent nightshifts. The thermic effect of feeding (ie, energy expenditure after food intake) was lower in response to late dinner on the first night shift. Subjective appetite decreased during nightshifts despite a decrease in levels of leptin and peptide-YY, another anorexigenic hormone. The combination of decreased energy expenditure and lower thermal effect of feeding after late meals could explain increased obesity in shift workers who often eat at night.

A final experimental study was designed to distinguish the effects of the behavioral cycles (sleep-wake, fasting-feeding, and activity), the endogenous circadian system, and circadian disruption on glucose metabolism.[42] The protocol involved 2 8-day crossover studies when the behavioral cycles were aligned or misaligned (12-hour shift) with their endogenous circadian system. Glucose tolerance was assessed at 8 AM and 8 PM in response to an identical mixed meal along with a measurement of lipids. Postprandial glucose levels were 17% higher in the biological evening than morning and the early phase postprandial insulin response was 27% lower in the evening, indicative of insufficient beta cell response. This endogenous circadian effect was much larger than that of the behavioral cycle effect (8% higher postprandial glucose and 14% lower insulin responses at dinner time compared with breakfast time). In addition, circadian misalignment (12-hour behavioral cycle inversion) increased postprandial glucose levels by 6% despite a 14% higher late-phase postprandial insulin response, suggesting reduced insulin sensitivity during misalignment. This study demonstrates the relative importance of the endogenous circadian system, the behavioral cycle, and circadian misalignment on glucose metabolism.

In summary, these experimental studies have demonstrated the importance of the circadian system and the timing of behaviors such as eating in controlling metabolism, and have provided insights into the mechanisms linking circadian disruption to increased cardiometabolic disease risk.

Circadian disruption contributes to increased cardiometabolic risks. Circadian misalignment results in

1. Impaired glucose tolerance as a result of decreased insulin sensitivity and inadequate beta cell response
2. Elevated inflammatory markers
3. Elevated mean arterial pressure
4. Decreased energy expenditure

OBSERVATIONAL STUDIES OF MILDER CIRCADIAN DISRUPTION

Shift work can be an extreme form of circadian disruption but circadian disruption in milder forms

Table 1
Circadian disruption experiments in healthy volunteers with evaluation of cardiometabolic changes

Study	Number of Subjects	Protocol	Assessments[a]	Results
Scheer et al,[38] 2009	10	10-d forced desynchrony protocol of 28-h day, consisted of 2 baseline days (8-h habitual sleep) followed by 7 recurring 28-h sleep-wake cycles under dim light conditions, with 4 isocaloric meals during each cycle. Ratio of scheduled sleep to wake was maintained at 1:2	• Hourly sample of plasma leptin, insulin, glucose, cortisol • Blood pressure	During circadian misalignment (subjects ate and slept 12 h from their habitual time): • Leptin decreased by 17% • Glucose increased by 6% (from postprandial rather than fasting levels) and insulin increased by 22%, suggesting decreased insulin sensitivity and insufficient pancreatic beta cell response • Mean arterial pressure increased by 3 mm Hg during wakefulness • Reversal of daily cortisol rhythm
Buxton et al,[39] 2012	21 (11 mean age 23 y, 10 mean age 60 y)	3 wk of forced desynchrony (28-h day) with 5.6-h/24 h sleep restriction, followed by 9 recovery days (24-h) with 10-h sleep opportunity/d	• Glucose and insulin response to standardized breakfast • RMR • 24-h profile of leptin and free ghrelin	At the end of concurrent sleep restriction and circadian disruption: • Glucose levels increased, both fasting (by 8%) and postprandial (by 14%); these returned to baseline after 9-d recovery period • Decreased fasting and postprandial peak insulin levels, reflecting inadequate pancreatic beta cell function • RMR decreased by 8% • Leptin profiled slightly decreased and free ghrelin profile slightly increased; these also occurred during recovery compared with baseline • Overall, no significant differences in these metabolic changes between younger and older participants
Leproult et al,[40] 2014	26 (19 male)	A parallel design comparing 8-d of sleep restriction (5 h) and sleep restriction combined with circadian misalignment (5-h bedtime with 8.5 sleep onset delayed for 4 of 8 d)	• Intravenous glucose tolerance test at baseline and the end of the experiment • Inflammatory marker hs-CRP measurement	At the end of the experiment: • Insulin sensitivity decreased from baseline in both circadian aligned and misaligned groups; this was not compensated by increased beta cell response • Men in the misaligned group had twice as large reduction in insulin sensitivity compared with the aligned group; differences in women were not apparent possibly due to small number of participants • hs-CRP increased significantly in misaligned group; in men, the misaligned group had levels more than doubled those of aligned group

McHill et al,[41] 2014	14	6-d inpatient simulated nightshift protocol (3-d daytime schedule followed by 3-d nightshift schedule), conducted in a whole-room calorimeter	• EE • Energy expenditure after meal (TEF) • Macronutrient use • Appetite rating, leptin, peptide-YY and ghrelin	During nightshifts: • EE decreased by 3% • TEF decreased in response to late dinner on first nightshift • Total fat use increased, and carbohydrate and protein use decreased • Appetite rating was lower despite lower levels of leptin and peptide-YY; ghrelin was unchanged
Morris et al,[42] 2015	14	Two 8 d of circadian aligned and circadian misaligned to evaluate the relative effects of behavioral cycle, endogenous circadian system and circadian misalignment on glucose and lipids metabolism	• Glucose, insulin and FFA responses to standard mixed meal test at 8 AM and 8 PM	• Postprandial glucose was 17% higher in the biological evening than morning, with 27% reduction in early phase postprandial insulin response, indicative of insufficient beta cell response • These changes were larger than the effects of the behavioral cycle • Circadian misalignment resulted in reduced glucose tolerance with increased later-phase insulin secretion, suggesting increased insulin resistance • FFA higher before dinner than breakfast time, and higher during circadian misalignment

Abbreviations: EE, total daily expenditure; FFA, free fatty acid; hs-CRP, high-sensitivity C-reactive protein; RMR, resting metabolic rate; TEF, thermal effect of feeding.

[a] Some studies had additional assessments. Please refer to references listed.

can also be detrimental. For example, going to bed at a different time on work or school days than on free days or weekends can lead to social jet lag, which may also be associated with cardiometabolic function. Also, the clock time that someone goes to bed, which can be a measure of chronotype, may be associated with cardiometabolic function. Finally, the time of day someone prefers to sleep versus be active, often called circadian preference, may be another characteristic of chronotype associated with cardiometabolic health. In this section, the association between cardiometabolic function and social jet lag and chronotype is discussed.

Many individuals in modern society experience social jet lag because of obligations such as work or school that require a specific wake time, and this obligation is lifted on free days.[43] In a large epidemiologic survey of more than 65,000 participants, greater social jet lag was associated with being overweight (BMI $\geq$25 kg/m^2).[44] In addition, among overweight participants, there was a positive correlation between social jet lag and BMI; those who slept at a later clock time had a higher BMI. Subsequent studies have demonstrated an association between social jet lag and adverse cardiometabolic profiles. In a study of 145 healthy participants, those with a social jet lag greater than or equal to 2 hours had significantly higher fasting morning cortisol and higher area-under-the-curve of cortisol levels collected over 5 hours starting in the morning.[45] Those with a social jet lag greater than or equal to 2 hours also had higher resting heart rate, shorter average sleep duration, and less physical activity. In a larger study of 815 non–shift workers, participants with greater social jet lag were more likely to be obese (OR 1.2, 95% CI 1.0–1.5) and to have the metabolic syndrome (OR 1.3, 95% CI 1.0–1.6).[46] Furthermore, among those who were obese and had the metabolic syndrome, greater social jet lag was also associated with an increased odds of having elevated glycated hemoglobin ($\geq$5.7%) and elevated inflammation (hs-CRP levels>3 mg/L).[46]

Individuals with a later chronotype, that is, those who sleep at a later clock time, often have a greater degree of circadian misalignment between behavioral rhythms and the endogenous central circadian clock, and they also often have greater social jet lag.[43] A later (evening) circadian preference and later chronotype have been associated with several cardiometabolic disorders and unhealthy behaviors (**Table 2**). In adolescents, large population studies have shown that those with evening circadian preference or later bed and wake times had a higher BMI z score, increased risk of being obese (OR 2.16), and less time spent

in moderate-to-vigorous physical activity.[47,48] An unhealthy diet may partly play a role in this association because those with evening preference were reported to have worse dietary habits, including frequent snacking, less fruits and vegetables consumption, increased caloric intake from fat, and meal skipping.[48–51] In an 8-week prospective study of 159 college freshmen, students who were evening types gained more weight than those who were morning types.[52]

In addition to obesity, having a later chronotype is also associated with increased cardiovascular risk. For example, obese short sleepers with an evening chronotype had higher stress hormone levels (24-hour urinary epinephrine and plasma corticotropin levels) and higher resting heart rates.[51] Two large population-based studies of more than 6000 participants revealed that evening chronotype was associated with increased odds of having type 2 diabetes (OR 1.73[53] and 2.5 in men and women combined[54]). Evening chronotype was also associated with increased odds of having arterial hypertension (OR 1.3).[54] In addition, in a clinic-based study of 194 subjects with type 2 diabetes, later chronotype based on bedtimes was associated with poorer glycemic control independently of sleep duration.[55] Subsequent studies in type 2 diabetes subjects (total 826 participants) have confirmed the association between evening chronotype and poorer glycemic control.[56,57] Evening chronotype in type 2 diabetes subjects was also associated with higher triglycerides and lower HDL levels.[57]

These studies suggest that milder forms of circadian disruption, not just the more extreme circadian disruption observed in shift workers, are associated with adverse cardiometabolic function. Future research should explore whether interventions to reduce circadian disruption and/or advancing bedtimes can improve cardiometabolic health.

POTENTIAL MEDIATORS LINKING EVENING CHRONOTYPE OR SHIFT WORK AND CARDIOMETABOLIC DISEASE

There are a few potential mediators linking evening chronotype and shift work to circadian disruption and ultimately to cardiometabolic disease (**Fig. 1**). These include reduced sleep duration or quality, inappropriate timing of meals, and light at night. These potential mediators and their associations with cardiometabolic disease are briefly reviewed.

Sleep

Chronotype and shift work is often associated with reduced sleep duration and quality.[16,45] Previous research has demonstrated that inadequate sleep durations, including short sleep, as well as poorer sleep quality are associated with cardiometabolic disease. Several meta-analyses of existing studies found that short sleep is associated with increased odds of prevalent obesity,[58] prevalent metabolic syndrome,[59] prevalent hypertension,[60] incident type 2 diabetes,[61] incident hypertension in those less than 65 years old,[60] and increased risk of developing or dying of coronary heart disease (CHD).[62] Furthermore, poor sleep quality has also been associated with increased risk of incident type 2 diabetes.[61] The association between sleep and cardiometabolic disease has been reviewed extensively.[63,64] Thus, impairments in sleep could partially mediate the association between shift work or chronotype and cardiometabolic disease.

Meal Timing

The timing of meals can affect internal circadian alignment because food metabolites serve as synchronizing signals for the clocks in many peripheral tissues and organs.[65] Exposure to food at an inappropriate time of day could lead to misalignment between central and peripheral clocks, which could impair metabolism and lead to weight gain.[66] Indeed, in an experimental model, mice fed at the wrong time of day gained more weight than mice with access to food at the appropriate circadian time despite similar food intake and physical activity.[67]

Studies in humans have also observed a relationship between meal timing and altered metabolism. A randomized crossover study in 32 women compared the effects of eating an early lunch (13:00) to a late lunch (16:30). Compared with the early lunch, the late lunch was associated with decreased pre-meal resting-energy expenditure, decreased pre-meal carbohydrate oxidation, decreased thermal effect of food, as well as decreased glucose tolerance to meal.[68] Decreased energy expenditure and decreased glucose tolerance are risk factors for weight gain and diabetes and, therefore, these results provide evidence for a link between eating at a later clock time and metabolic disease. Another study found that more calories consumed after 20:00 was associated with higher BMI, even after controlling for sleep timing and duration.[69] Studies of weight loss interventions have also demonstrated the importance of timing of food intake. In a 20-week weight loss study of 420 participants, those who consumed their main meal (lunch in this Mediterranean population) before 15:00 lost 2.2 kg more on average than those who ate after 15:00, despite consuming similar amount of calories.[70] In a second weight loss study, women were randomized to either a large proportion of calories earlier in

the day (70% for breakfast, morning snack, and lunch and 30% for afternoon snack and dinner) or a more even distribution (55% for breakfast through lunch and 45% for afternoon snack and dinner) for 3 months.[71] Those who eat more food earlier in the day lost significantly more weight (−8.2 vs −6.5 kg, $P = .028$), reduced waist circumference by more (−7 vs −5 cm, $P = .033$), lost more fat mass (−6.8 vs −4.5 kg, $P = .031$), and improved their insulin sensitivity more. A qualitative study found that a strategy used by individuals who maintained 10% weight loss for at least 1 year was eating a small dinner, a strategy not used by individuals who regained weight after an initial loss.[72] Finally, because glucose tolerance is known to be worse in the evening,[73] late eating may also affect glycemic control in patients with diabetes. In fact, a study of patients with type 2 diabetes demonstrated that a greater amount of daily calories consumed at dinner was associated with poorer glycemic control, independently of chronotype.[55] Interestingly, a recent randomized crossover study in type 2 diabetes patients compared a hypoenergetic diet of 2 larger meals (breakfast and lunch) to 6 smaller meals in 54 patients for 12 weeks. Two larger meals resulted in a significantly greater reduction in body weight, liver fat content, fasting plasma glucose, C-peptide, and glucagon, and higher insulin sensitivity, than the same caloric restriction split into 6 meals,[74] indicating the timing of food intake has an important effect on metabolism.

Another potentially important meal pattern is breakfast skipping. There is overwhelming evidence that breakfast skipping is detrimental to health, including higher risks of overweight and obesity, increased visceral adiposity, insulin resistance, type 2 diabetes, and dyslipidemia. For example, a longitudinal study of 2184 participants over 20 years found that those who skipped breakfast in both childhood and adulthood had significantly greater waist circumference and higher fasting insulin, total cholesterol, and low-density lipoprotein cholesterol than those who consumed breakfast at both time points.[75] A study of 3598 participants from the community-based Coronary Artery Risk Development in Young Adults (CARDIA) study found that, relative to those with infrequent breakfast consumption (0–3 days/week), participants who reported eating breakfast daily gained 1.9 kg less weight over 18 years ($P = .001$), along with significant reduction in the incidence of obesity, metabolic syndrome, and hypertension.[76] Moreover, in a cohort of 26,902 American men, those who skipped breakfast had a 27% higher risk of CHD compared with men who did not.[77] In addition

Table 2
Studies of the associations between chronotype and metabolic outcomes

Study	Population	Number of Subjects	Chronotype Assessments	Metabolic Outcomes
Arora & Taheri,[48] 2015	Young adolescents (aged 11–13 y)	511	Morningness-eveningness questionnaire	• Evening chronotype was associated with higher BMI z score than morning chronotype • Later chronotype was associated with unhealthy diet (snacks, night-time caffeine, and inadequate fruits and vegetables consumption)
Olds et al,[47] 2011	Adolescent (aged 9–16 y)	2200	Bedtime and wake time Participants categorized into: Early-bed, early-rise Early-bed, late-rise Late-bed, early-rise Late-bed, late-rise	• Late-bed, late-rise participants had more screen time by 48 min/d and 27 min less moderate-to-vigorous physical activity than early-bed, early-rise, despite similar sleep duration • Late-bed, late-rise participants had higher BMI z score and were 2.16 times more likely to be obese compared with early-bed, early-rise
Sato-Mito et al,[49] 2011	Young adults (aged 18–20 y)	3304	Midpoint of sleep	• Late midpoint of sleep negatively correlated with unhealthy dietary habits, including increased caloric intake from alcohol and fat with decreased protein and vitamins and minerals consumption • Late midpoint of sleep was associated with meal skipping and watching TV at mealtime
Culnan et al,[52] 2013	College freshmen (mean age 18 y)	159	Morningness-eveningness questionnaire	• Evening types had significantly more BMI gain at 8 wk follow-up compared with morning type
Lucassen et al,[51] 2013	Obese adults with <6.5 h of sleep	119	Morningness-eveningness questionnaire	• Eveningness was associated with fewer and larger meals, lower HDL cholesterol, more sleep apnea and higher stress hormones (24-h urinary epinephrine and morning plasma corticotropin), and higher morning resting heart rate

Study	Population	N	Measure	Findings
Nakanishi-Minami et al,[94] 2012	Adults	32 healthy, and 74 T2DM	Bedtime and wake time	• T2DM patients had significantly later bedtime on weekdays and weekends (by 49 and 68 min, respectively) than those without diabetes • T2DM patients woke up significantly later than those without diabetes, by 31 min on weekdays and 34 min on weekends
Merikanto et al,[54] 2013	Adults, aged 25–74 y	4589	Modified Morningness-eveningness questionnaire	• Evening types had increased risk of having T2DM (2.5-fold) and arterial hypertension (1.3-fold)
Yu et al,[53] 2015	Adults, aged 47–59 y	1620	Morningness-eveningness questionnaire	• Men with evening types had increased risk of having diabetes (OR 2.98) • Women with evening types had increased risk of having metabolic syndrome (OR 1.74)
Reutrakul et al,[55] 2013	Adults with T2DM	194	Mid sleep time on free day corrected for sleep debt	• Later chronotype was independently associated with poorer glycemic control; the association was partially mediated by greater percentage of total daily calories consumed at dinner
Iwasaki et al,[56] 2013	Adults with T2DM	101	Morningness-eveningness questionnaire	• More evening preference was associated with poorer glycemic control (hemoglobin A1c levels) and poorer sleep quality
Osonoi et al,[57] 2014	Adults with T2DM	725	Morningness-eveningness questionnaire	• Eveningness was associated with poorer glycemic control, higher triglycerides, and lower HDL cholesterol levels

Abbreviation: T2DM, type 2 diabetes.

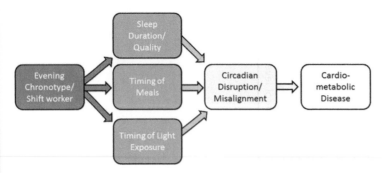

Fig. 1. Potential pathways leading from later chronotype or shift work to circadian disruption and cardiometabolic disease.

men who ate after going to bed had a 55% higher CHD risk than men who did not. However, once adjusting for health factors, such as BMI, hypertension, hypercholesterolemia, and diabetes status, the associations were no longer significant. Another longitudinal study of 29,206 men reported that breakfast skipping was associated with a 21% increase in risk of developing type 2 diabetes, even after adjustment for BMI[78] and the Nurses' Health Study of women also observed a significant association between breakfast skipping and incident diabetes.[79] A recent meta-analysis of 106,935 participants found that breakfast skipping was associated with type 2 diabetes.[34,80] In addition, in patients with type 2 diabetes, breakfast skipping was found to be associated with poorer glycemic control.[50,81,82] A recent study in Japan examined the combination of breakfast skipping and late-night eating and found that a combination of breakfast skipping and late-night eating (consumed dinner within 2 hours of bedtime ≥3 times/week) was associated with the presence of the metabolic syndrome (OR 1.17), whereas breakfast skipping or late-night eating alone was not.[83] Finally, a weight-loss intervention study found that eating breakfast was associated with greater weight loss despite similar caloric restriction[84] but a second intervention study found no effect of breakfast eating recommendations.[85]

Overall, the evidence suggests a relationship between meal timing or daily food distribution and cardiometabolic risk. Although breakfast skipping and eating at night are associated with adverse cardiometabolic profiles, more interventional studies are needed to demonstrate whether manipulating meal timing will result in improved metabolism.

Light at Night

Another potential mediator between late chronotype or shift work and cardiometabolic disease is exposure to artificial light at night. Light is the primary synchronizer of the central circadian clock and, therefore, exposure to light during the

biological night could lead to circadian disruption. There is some evidence from animal studies that exposure to light at night can impair metabolism. In these studies, male mice that were exposed to a high fat diet and dim light at night had increased weight gain, reduced glucose tolerance, and altered insulin secretion compared with mice that were not exposed to light at night, despite equivalent caloric intake.[86] Furthermore, the timing of the food intake was shifted when exposed to light,[87] indicating that animals exposed to light at night may also be eating more food at an inappropriate circadian time.

Another mechanism through which light at night could impair cardiometabolic function is through melatonin. Melatonin is a hormone primarily secreted by the pineal gland and its release is suppressed by light. Melatonin plays an important role in circadian physiology[88] and also plays a role in sleep promotion.[89] More recently, melatonin has been recognized as playing an important role in metabolism.[90,91] Lower melatonin levels were associated with increased risk of incident diabetes in a large cohort study.[92] Thus, individuals who stay up later will be exposed to more artificial light, which will suppress melatonin and potentially reduce the total amount of melatonin secreted, putting them at risk of diabetes.

The role artificial light may play in health was recently recognized by the American Medical Association (AMA). In June, 2012, the AMA House of Delegates adopted a policy statement on nighttime lighting. The Executive Summary states, "Other diseases that may be exacerbated by circadian disruption include obesity, diabetes…"[93] Thus, there is recognition that electric light could lead to circadian disruption, which, in turn, could impair human health.

SUMMARY

Circadian disruption is associated with impairments in cardiometabolic function and increased risk of obesity, diabetes, and CVD. This association is not only among the most severe forms of circadian disruption (ie, shift work), but is also observed with milder delays in the timing of sleep and meals. Future research should determine whether manipulating the timing of sleep, meals, or light exposure can help to improve cardiometabolic health.

REFERENCES

1. Swinburn BA, Sacks G, Hall KD, et al. The global obesity pandemic: shaped by global drivers and local environments. Lancet 2011;378(9793):804–14.
2. Seidell J. Obesity, insulin resistance and diabetes–a worldwide epidemic. Br J Nutr 2000;83(Suppl 1): S5–8.
3. Ettaro L, Songer TJ, Zhang P, et al. Cost-of-illness studies in diabetes mellitus. Pharmacoeconomics 2004;22(3):149–64.
4. Franco OH, Steyerberg EW, Hu FB, et al. Associations of diabetes mellitus with total life expectancy and life expectancy with and without cardiovascular disease. Arch Intern Med 2007;167(11):1145–51.
5. Solomon CG, Manson JE. Obesity and mortality: a review of the epidemiologic data. Am J Clin Nutr 1997;66(4 Suppl):1044S–50S.
6. Wolf AM, Colditz GA. Current estimates of the economic cost of obesity in the United States. Obes Res 1998;6(2):97–106.
7. Brown DL, Feskanich D, Sánchez BN, et al. Rotating night shift work and the risk of ischemic stroke. Am J Epidemiol 2009;169(11):1370–7.
8. Kawachi I, Colditz GA, Stampfer MJ, et al. Prospective study of shift work and risk of coronary heart disease in women. Circulation 1995;92(11):3178–82.
9. Knutsson A, Akerstedt T, Jonsson BG, et al. Increased risk of ischaemic heart disease in shift workers. Lancet 1986;2:89–92.
10. Sakata K, Suwazono Y, Harada H, et al. The relationship between shift work and the onset of hypertension in male Japanese workers. J Occup Environ Med 2003;45(9):1002–6.
11. Marqueze EC, Ulhoa MA, Moreno CR. Effects of irregular-shift work and physical activity on cardiovascular risk factors in truck drivers. Rev Saude Publica 2013;47(3):497–505.
12. Ha M, Park J. Shiftwork and metabolic risk factors of cardiovascular disease. J Occup Health 2005;47(2): 89–95.
13. Amir O, Alroy S, Schliamser JE, et al. Brachial artery endothelial function in residents and fellows working night shifts. Am J Cardiol 2004;93(7):947–9.
14. Murata K, Yano E, Hashimoto H, et al. Effects of shift work on QTc interval and blood pressure in relation to heart rate variability. Int Arch Occup Environ Health 2005;78(4):287–92.
15. Eriksson AK, van den Donk M, Hilding A, et al. Work stress, sense of coherence, and risk of type 2 diabetes in a prospective study of middle-aged Swedish men and women. Diabetes Care 2013;36(9): 2683–9.
16. Pan A, Schernhammer ES, Sun Q, et al. Rotating night shift work and risk of type 2 diabetes: two prospective cohort studies in women. PLoS Med 2011; 8(12):e1001141.
17. Kroenke CH, Spiegelman D, Manson J, et al. Work characteristics and incidence of type 2 diabetes in women. Am J Epidemiol 2007;165(2):175–83.
18. Gan Y, Yang C, Tong X, et al. Shift work and diabetes mellitus: a meta-analysis of observational studies. Occup Environ Med 2015;72(1):72–8.
19. Morikawa Y, Nakagawa H, Miura K, et al. Effect of shift work on body mass index and metabolic parameters. Scand J Work Environ Health 2007;33(1):45–50.
20. Barbadoro P, Santarelli L, Croce N, et al. Rotating shift-work as an independent risk factor for overweight Italian workers: a cross-sectional study. PLoS One 2013;8(5):e63289.
21. van Amelsvoort L, Schouten E, Kok F. Duration of shiftwork related to body mass index and waist to hip ratio. Int J Obes 1999;23:973–8.
22. Nakamura K, Shimai S, Kikuchi S, et al. Shift work and risk factors for coronary heart disease in Japanese blue-collar workers: serum lipids and anthropometric characteristics. Occup Med (Lond) 1997; 47(3):142–6.
23. Kim MJ, Son KH, Park HY, et al. Association between shift work and obesity among female nurses: Korean Nurses' Survey. BMC Public Health 2013;13:1204.
24. Karlsson B, Knutsson A, Lindahl B. Is there an association between shift work and having a metabolic syndrome? Results from a population based study of 27,485 people. Occup Environ Med 2001;58(11): 747–52.
25. Romon M, Nuttens MC, Fievet C, et al. Increased triglyceride levels in shift workers. Am J Med 1992; 93(3):259–62.
26. Dochi M, Suwazono Y, Sakata K, et al. Shift work is a risk factor for increased total cholesterol level: a 14-year prospective cohort study in 6886 male workers. Occup Environ Med 2009;66(9):592–7.
27. Knutsson A, Akerstedt T, Jonsson BG. Prevalence of risk factors for coronary artery disease among day and shift workers. Scand J Work Environ Health 1988;14(5):317–21.
28. Karlsson BH, Knutsson AK, Lindahl BO, et al. Metabolic disturbances in male workers with rotating three-shift work. Results of the WOLF study. Int Arch Occup Environ Health 2003;76(6):424–30.
29. Nagaya T, Yoshida H, Takahashi H, et al. Markers of insulin resistance in day and shift workers aged 30-59 years. Int Arch Occup Environ Health 2002;75(8): 562–8.

30. Esquirol Y, Bongard V, Ferrieres J, et al. Shiftwork and higher pancreatic secretion: early detection of an intermediate state of insulin resistance? Chronobiol Int 2012;29(9):1258–66.

31. Kawada T, Otsuka T. Effect of shift work on the development of metabolic syndrome after 3 years in Japanese male workers. Arch Environ Occup Health 2014;69(1):55–61.

32. De Bacquer D, Van Risseghem M, Clays E, et al. Rotating shift work and the metabolic syndrome: a prospective study. Int J Epidemiol 2009;38(3):848–54.

33. Lin YC, Hsiao TJ, Chen PC. Persistent rotating shift-work exposure accelerates development of metabolic syndrome among middle-aged female employees: a five-year follow-up. Chronobiol Int 2009;26(4):740–55.

34. Boggild H, Suadicani P, Hein HO, et al. Shift work, social class, and ischaemic heart disease in middle aged and elderly men; a 22 year follow up in the Copenhagen Male Study. Occup Environ Med 1999; 56(9):640–5.

35. Bursey RG. A cardiovascular study of shift workers with respect to coronary artery disease risk factor prevalence. J Soc Occup Med 1990; 40(2):65–7.

36. Fouriaud C, Jacquinet-Salord MC, Degoulet P, et al. Influence of socioprofessional conditions on blood pressure levels and hypertension control. Epidemiologic study of 6,665 subjects in the Paris district. Am J Epidemiol 1984;120(1):72–86.

37. Ika K, Suzuki E, Mitsuhashi T, et al. Shift work and diabetes mellitus among male workers in Japan: does the intensity of shift work matter? Acta Med Okayama 2013;67(1):25–33.

38. Scheer FA, Hilton MF, Mantzoros CS, et al. Adverse metabolic and cardiovascular consequences of circadian misalignment. Proc Natl Acad Sci U S A 2009;106(11):4453–8.

39. Buxton OM, Cain SW, O'Connor SP, et al. Adverse metabolic consequences in humans of prolonged sleep restriction combined with circadian disruption. Sci Transl Med 2012;4(129):129ra43.

40. Leproult R, Holmback U, Van Cauter E. Circadian misalignment augments markers of insulin resistance and inflammation, independently of sleep loss. Diabetes 2014;63(6):1860–9.

41. McHill AW, Melanson EL, Higgins J, et al. Impact of circadian misalignment on energy metabolism during simulated nightshift work. Proc Natl Acad Sci U S A 2014;111(48):17302–7.

42. Morris CJ, Yang JN, Garcia JI, et al. Endogenous circadian system and circadian misalignment impact glucose tolerance via separate mechanisms in humans. Proc Natl Acad Sci U S A 2015;112(17): E2225–34.

43. Wittmann M, Dinich J, Merrow M, et al. Social jetlag: misalignment of biological and social time. Chronobiol Int 2006;23(1–2):497–509.

44. Roenneberg T, Allebrandt KV, Merrow M, et al. Social jetlag and obesity. Curr Biol 2012;22(10): 939–43.

45. Rutters F, Lemmens SG, Adam TC, et al. Is social jetlag associated with an adverse endocrine, behavioral, and cardiovascular risk profile? J Biol Rhythms 2014; 29(5):377–83.

46. Parsons MJ, Moffitt TE, Gregory AM, et al. Social jetlag, obesity and metabolic disorder: investigation in a cohort study. Int J Obes (Lond) 2015; 39(5):842–8.

47. Olds TS, Maher CA, Matricciani L. Sleep duration or bedtime? Exploring the relationship between sleep habits and weight status and activity patterns. Sleep 2011;34(10):1299–307.

48. Arora T, Taheri S. Associations among late chronotype, body mass index and dietary behaviors in young adolescents. Int J Obes (Lond) 2015;39(1): 39–44.

49. Sato-Mito N, Sasaki S, Murakami K, et al. The midpoint of sleep is associated with dietary intake and dietary behavior among young Japanese women. Sleep Med 2011;12(3):289–94.

50. Reutrakul S, Hood MM, Crowley SJ, et al. The relationship between breakfast skipping, chronotype, and glycemic control in type 2 diabetes. Chronobiol Int 2014;31(1):64–71.

51. Lucassen EA, Zhao X, Rother KI, et al. Evening chronotype is associated with changes in eating behavior, more sleep apnea, and increased stress hormones in short sleeping obese individuals. PLoS One 2013;8(3):e56519.

52. Culnan E, Kloss JD, Grandner M. A prospective study of weight gain associated with chronotype among college freshmen. Chronobiol Int 2013; 30(5):682–90.

53. Yu JH, Yun CH, Ahn JH, et al. Evening chronotype is associated with metabolic disorders and body composition in middle-aged adults. J Clin Endocrinol Metab 2015;100(4):1494–502.

54. Merikanto I, Lahti T, Puolijoki H, et al. Associations of chronotype and sleep with cardiovascular diseases and type 2 diabetes. Chronobiol Int 2013;30(4): 470–7.

55. Reutrakul S, Hood MM, Crowley SJ, et al. Chronotype is independently associated with glycemic control in type 2 diabetes. Diabetes Care 2013;36(9): 2523–9.

56. Iwasaki M, Hirose T, Mita T, et al. Morningness-eveningness questionnaire score correlates with glycated hemoglobin in middle-aged male workers with type 2 diabetes mellitus. J Diabetes Investig 2013;4(4):376–81.

57. Osonoi Y, Mita T, Osonoi T, et al. Morningness-eveningness questionnaire score and metabolic parameters in patients with type 2 diabetes mellitus. Chronobiol Int 2014;31(9):1017–23.

58. Cappuccio FP, Taggart FM, Kandala NB, et al. Meta-analysis of short sleep duration and obesity in children and adults. Sleep 2008;31(5):619–26.

59. Ju SY, Choi WS. Sleep duration and metabolic syndrome in adult populations: a meta-analysis of observational studies. Nutr Diabetes 2013;3:e65.

60. Wang Q, Xi B, Liu M, et al. Short sleep duration is associated with hypertension risk among adults: a systematic review and meta-analysis. Hypertens Res 2012;35(10):1012–8.

61. Cappuccio FP, D'Elia L, Strazzullo P, et al. Quantity and quality of sleep and incidence of type 2 diabetes: a systematic review and meta-analysis. Diabetes Care 2010;33(2):414–20.

62. Cappuccio FP, Cooper D, D'Elia L, et al. Sleep duration predicts cardiovascular outcomes: a systematic review and meta-analysis of prospective studies. Eur Heart J 2011;32(12):1484–92.

63. Ip M, Mokhlesi B. Sleep and Glucose Intolerance/Diabetes Mellitus. Sleep Med Clin 2007;2:19–29.

64. Knutson KL. Does inadequate sleep play a role in vulnerability to obesity? Am J Hum Biol 2012;24:361–71.

65. Dibner C, Schibler U, Albrecht U. The mammalian circadian timing system: organization and coordination of central and peripheral clocks. Annu Rev Physiol 2010;72:517–49.

66. Garaulet M, Gomez-Abellan P. Timing of food intake and obesity: a novel association. Physiol Behav 2014;134:44–50.

67. Arble DM, Bass J, Laposky AD, et al. Circadian timing of food intake contributes to weight gain. Obesity (Silver Spring) 2009;17(11):2100–2.

68. Bandin C, Scheer FA, Luque AJ, et al. Meal timing affects glucose tolerance, substrate oxidation and circadian-related variables: a randomized, crossover trial. Int J Obes (Lond) 2015;39(5):828–33.

69. Baron KG, Reid KJ, Kern AS, et al. Role of sleep timing in caloric intake and BMI. Obesity (Silver Spring) 2011;19(7):1374–81.

70. Garaulet M, Gómez-Abellán P, Alburquerque-Béjar JJ, et al. Timing of food intake predicts weight loss effectiveness. Int J Obes (Lond) 2013;37(4):604–11.

71. Lombardo M, Bellia A, Padua E, et al. Morning meal more efficient for fat loss in a 3-month lifestyle intervention. J Am Coll Nutr 2014;33(3):198–205.

72. Karfopoulou E, Mouliou K, Koutras Y, et al. Behaviours associated with weight loss maintenance and regaining in a Mediterranean population sample. A qualitative study. Clin Obes 2013;3(5):141–9.

73. Van Cauter E, Polonsky KS, Scheen AJ. Roles of circadian rhythmicity and sleep in human glucose regulation. Endocr Rev 1997;18:716–38.

74. Kahleova H, Belinova L, Malinska H, et al. Eating two larger meals a day (breakfast and lunch) is more effective than six smaller meals in a reduced-energy regimen for patients with type 2 diabetes: a randomised crossover study. Diabetologia 2014;57(8):1552–60.

75. Smith KJ, Gall SL, McNaughton SA, et al. Skipping breakfast: longitudinal associations with cardiometabolic risk factors in the childhood determinants of adult health Study. Am J Clin Nutr 2010;92(6):1316–25.

76. Odegaard AO, Jacobs DR Jr, Steffen LM, et al. Breakfast frequency and development of metabolic risk. Diabetes Care 2013;36(10):3100–6.

77. Cahill LE, Chiuve SE, Mekary RA, et al. Prospective study of breakfast eating and incident coronary heart disease in a cohort of male US health professionals. Circulation 2013;128(4):337–43.

78. Mekary RA, Giovannucci E, Willett WC, et al. Eating patterns and type 2 diabetes risk in men: breakfast omission, eating frequency, and snacking. Am J Clin Nutr 2012;95(5):1182–9.

79. Mekary RA, Giovannucci E, Cahill L, et al. Eating patterns and type 2 diabetes risk in older women: breakfast consumption and eating frequency. Am J Clin Nutr 2013;98(2):436–43.

80. Bi H, Gan Y, Yang C, et al. Breakfast skipping and the risk of type 2 diabetes: a meta-analysis of observational studies. Public Health Nutr 2015;1–7.

81. Kollannoor-Samuel G, Chhabra J, Fernandez ML, et al. Determinants of fasting plasma glucose and glycosylated hemoglobin among low income Latinos with poorly controlled type 2 diabetes. J Immigr Minor Health 2011;13(5):809–17.

82. Schmidt LE, Rost KM, McGill JB, et al. The relationship between eating patterns and metabolic control in patients with non-insulin-dependent diabetes mellitus (NIDDM). Diabetes Educ 1994;20(4):317–21.

83. Kutsuma A, Nakajima K, Suwa K. Potential association between breakfast skipping and Concomitant late-night-dinner eating with metabolic syndrome and proteinuria in the Japanese population. Scientifica (Cairo) 2014;2014:253581.

84. Schlundt DG, Hill JO, Sbrocco T, et al. The role of breakfast in the treatment of obesity: a randomized clinical trial. Am J Clin Nutr 1992;55(3):645–51.

85. Dhurandhar EJ, Dawson J, Alcorn A, et al. The effectiveness of breakfast recommendations on weight loss: a randomized controlled trial. Am J Clin Nutr 2014;100(2):507–13.

86. Fonken LK, Lieberman RA, Weil ZM, et al. Dim light at night exaggerates weight gain and inflammation associated with a high-fat diet in male mice. Endocrinology 2013;154(10):3817–25.

87. Fonken LK, Workman JL, Walton JC, et al. Light at night increases body mass by shifting the time of food intake. Proc Natl Acad Sci U S A 2010;107(43):18664–9.

88. Emens JS, Burgess HJ. Effect of Light and Melatonin and Other Melatonin Receptor Agonists on Human Circadian Physiology. Sleep Med Clin 2015, in press.

89. Dubocovich ML. Melatonin receptors: role on sleep and circadian rhythm regulation. Sleep Med 2007; 8(Suppl 3):34–42.

90. Peschke E, Muhlbauer E. New evidence for a role of melatonin in glucose regulation. Best Pract Res Clin Endocrinol Metab 2010;24(5):829–41.

91. Acuna-Castroviejo D, Escames G, Venegas C, et al. Extrapineal melatonin: sources, regulation, and potential functions. Cell Mol Life Sci 2014;71(16): 2997–3025.

92. McMullan CJ, Schernhammer ES, Rimm EB, et al. Melatonin secretion and the incidence of type 2 diabetes. JAMA 2013;309(13):1388–96.

93. Stevens RG, Brainard GC, Blask DE, et al. Adverse health effects of nighttime lighting: comments on American Medical Association policy statement. Am J Prev Med 2013;45(3):343–6.

94. Nakanishi-Minami T, Kishida K, Funahashi T, et al. Sleep-wake cycle irregularities in type 2 diabetics. Diabetol Metab Syndr 2012;4(1):18.

Consequences of Circadian Disruption on Neurologic Health

Aleksandar Videnovic, MD, MSc[a],*, Phyllis C. Zee, MD, PhD[b]

KEYWORDS

- Circadian • Sleep • Clock genes • Cerebrovascular • Stroke • Alzheimer • Parkinson • Huntington

KEY POINTS

- Numerous brain diseases show a clear rhythmicity of symptoms and its outcomes seem to be influenced by the time of day.
- Circadian rhythm dysfunction is common in neurodegenerative disorders such as Alzheimer, Parkinson, and Huntington diseases.
- Circadian disruption may be a significant risk factor for cerebrovascular and neurodegenerative disorders.
- The circadian system may be a novel diagnosis and therapeutic target for neurologic diseases.

INTRODUCTION

The relevance of circadian rhythms and time-keeping for human health has been increasingly recognized not only by sleep medicine but also by many other medical specialties. Twenty-four-hour diurnal fluctuations in symptom intensity, responsiveness to treatment modalities, and survival have been well documented. Important advances in circadian biology over the past several decades provide an opportunity to systematically investigate relationships between diseases, endogenous circadian rhythms, and exogenous influences. Many neurologic disorders show fluctuating rhythms of symptoms and responsiveness to therapies. This article outlines the available literature pertinent to circadian function in common neurologic disorders with an emphasis on cerebrovascular and neurodegenerative disorders.

CIRCADIAN DISRUPTION IN CEREBROVASCULAR DISEASE

Stroke is the third leading cause of death in the United States. Sleep disorders are common in people who have had strokes. Sleep dysfunction has also been repeatedly linked with cardiovascular and cerebrovascular insults and implicated in poststroke recovery. Although well recognized, the relationship between sleep, circadian disruption, and stroke is not fully understood. Sleep and circadian dysfunction may lead to vascular events through direct or indirect mechanisms. Sleep loss, sleep disordered breathing, and sleep-related movement disorders, such as restless legs syndrome and periodic limb movements disorder, may increase the risk of stroke, hypertension, and cardiovascular disorders.[1] Sleep loss itself seems to be an independent risk factor for cerebrovascular events, likely because of alterations in the autonomic nervous system and immune homeostasis.[2]

Emerging evidence suggests important effects that circadian homeostasis has on cerebrovascular health. Major cardiovascular parameters such as heart rate (HR), blood pressure (BP), and endothelial function, known to affect a wide range of cerebrovascular disorders, have intrinsic circadian properties. The onset of major cerebrovascular disorders frequently shows a unique diurnal

a Department of Neurology, Massachusetts General Hospital, Harvard Medical School, 165 Cambridge Street, Suite 600, Boston, MA 02114, USA; b Northwestern University Feinberg School of Medicine, Abbott Hall 11th Floor, 710 North Lake Shore Drive, Chicago, IL 60611, USA
* Corresponding author.
E-mail address: avidenovic@mgh.harvard.edu

Sleep Med Clin 10 (2015) 469–480
http://dx.doi.org/10.1016/j.jsmc.2015.08.004
1556-407X/15/$ – see front matter © 2015 Elsevier Inc. All rights reserved.

pattern. Both epidemiologic data and animal model data strongly point to circadian disruption as a risk factor for cerebrovascular disease.

Circadian Cardiovascular Rhythms

BP, HR, and baroreceptor sensitivity show robust physiologic oscillations over a 24-hour period.[3] Normally BP dips overnight, increases shortly before awakening, and reaches its maximum during midmorning hours. Individuals with nondipping BP pattern have less than 10% decline/increase in systolic BP and/or diastolic BP during sleep relative to their mean daytime BP levels. Nondipping BP rhythm is associated with cardiac ventricular hypertrophy, renal dysfunction, and alterations in the cerebral vasculature.[4] Individuals lacking the normal circadian rhythm of BP are therefore at increased risk for cerebrovascular events, which tend to occur in the early morning hours. Factors contributing to cerebrovascular insult, in particular ischemic events, follow a circadian pattern.

Circadian Variation in Stroke Onset

Diurnal variation in stroke onset has been reported in numerous studies, with higher frequency of stroke occurring in the morning.[5] Approximately 55% of all ischemic strokes, 34% of all hemorrhagic strokes, and 50% of all transient ischemic attacks occur between 06:00 and 12:00 hours.[6] Mortality from stroke remains high in strokes occurring in the morning hours.[7] Although stroke shows this clustering in the morning, some studies reported a bimodal distribution of stroke onset in hemorrhagic strokes with the second peak being in the afternoon.[8–12] The effects of recombinant tissue plasminogen activator treatment on outcomes have been independent of time of day of stroke onset.[13] Most investigations related to 24-hour patterns in stroke are centered on the time of day when stroke occurred, lacking relevant determinants of exogenous influences such as the rest/activity rhythm and other known risk factors.

Pathophysiologic factors that may explain a diurnal pattern of stroke onset include early morning increase in BP (so-called morning surge), increased platelet aggregation, and prothrombotic factors, as well as blunting of endothelial function in the morning hours. The peak level of circadian sympathetic activity also occurs in the morning, which along with the simultaneous increased activity of the renin-angiotensin-aldosterone activity influences the morning increase in BP and HR. Further, the propensity for rapid eye movement (REM) sleep increases in the early morning hours. This stage of sleep is associated with reduced coronary blood flow and increased occurrence of coronary spasm, which contributes to heightened sympathetic activity and increases in BP and HR. Primary sleep disorders, such as sleep disordered breathing, are additional causes, through repetitive intermittent overnight hypoxemia and sympathetic activation. Most of the available studies failed to show significant demographic and clinical differences between wake-up strokes and those occurring while awake.[5] Available studies have numerous methodological limitations, and better controlled prospective investigations are needed to distinguish between stoke present on awakening and those while awake. This distinction is important because these differences have potential implications for treatment.

Other circadian rhythms implicated in the pathophysiology of cerebrovascular disease include rhythms of plasma viscosity, blood flow volume, hematocrit, peripheral resistance, and platelet levels. Platelet numbers and aggregation both have rhythmicity, with peak number of platelets being in the afternoon. Platelet aggregation response to various stimuli tends to peak during the late night or early morning hours. Several factors within the coagulation pathways have their own circadian rhythms. For example, the peak activity of factor II remains in close correlation with the peak incidence of thromboembolic events.

Aside from circadian rhythms, cerebrovascular events are also linked with periodicities longer than circadian. For example, fibrinolysis has circaseptan (approximately 7-day) rhythm with the lowest amplitude of the rhythm on Monday and the peak between Tuesday and Thursday. This pattern mirrors that of thromoembolic events during the week. Similarly, circannual variations in cardiovascular parameters may affect the pathophysiology of vascular events.[14] Numerous studies reported 7-day and annual patterns in stroke onset. It is important to emphasize that many exogenous stressors affect the occurrence of cerebrovascular events, likely through complex interactions with endogenous circadian rhythms. These factors may include emotional stress, napping, physical activity, and medication schedules.

Clock Genes and Cardiovascular Function

Circadian transcription rhythms have been shown in 4% to 6% of protein coding genes in mouse heart and aorta.[15–17] Similar oscillations persist in endothelial and vascular smooth muscle cells as well as in human cardiomyocytes.[18–20] Recent investigations suggest a role of the nuclear receptor PPARγ in BP rhythm regulation, likely through its interactions with Bmal1, a major circadian clock gene. Cry1/2 genes have also been implicated in the development of hypertension.[21,22] Deletion of a core clock gene, Bmal1, in heart and endothelium results in arrhythmias and loss of diurnal BP oscillation.[23,24] Internal desynchronization between the central circadian pacemaker and local cardiovascular clocks has been shown to affect cardiac structure and the expression of cardiac clock genes.[25] This internal desynchronization may arise from disruption of physiologic sleep-wake cycles. The relationship between molecular regulation of circadian rhythms and cardiovascular disease is likely bidirectional because cardiac hypertrophy and aortic constriction attenuate expression of several core clock genes throughout the cardiovascular system.[26,27] Recent investigations have suggested that differential susceptibility to neuronal damage from an ischemic insult depends on the time of day when the insult occurs.[28] Although the mechanisms that underlie this susceptibility to ischemic damage remain unknown, the role of ERK, a mitogen-activated protein kinase molecule, and its neuroprotection against glutamate toxicity on suprachiasmatic nucleus (SCN) neurons has recently been implicated.[29] Further investigations directed to understanding how circadian biology affects cerebrovascular and cardiovascular disorders on cellular and molecular levels and vice versa are much needed.

CIRCADIAN RHYTHMS IN AGING AND NEURODEGENERATION

Aging is associated with changes in the circadian system. Age-related changes in circadian rhythmicity result in a reduced amplitude and period length of circadian rhythms, an increased intradaily variability, and a decreased interdaily stability of a rhythm.[30–36] The timing of the rhythm is disturbed as well, leading to changes in the time relationship of rhythms to each other, known as internal desynchronization. This loss of coordination has negative consequences on rest-activity cycles and other physiologic and behavioral functions.[37] Numerous studies in humans have shown reduced amplitudes of melatonin rhythms, and phase advance of body temperature and melatonin with aging.[32,38–40] The circadian profile of cortisol in the elderly shows higher plasma levels at night, which results in an increased 24-hour mean cortisol level and a reduction in the rhythm amplitude.[40,41] These changes in circadian rhythmicity of cortisol secretion have been associated with cognitive impairments and increased propensity for awakenings with aging.[42–45] However, not all studies show age-related decline in the amplitude of the circadian markers.[46–48] This finding may be caused by several shortcomings, including small sample size, subject selection criteria, complex

medication regimens, and absence of well-controlled experimental conditions (ie, constant routine). Clearly the human data are inadequate and further studies are warranted.

Disrupted rest/activity cycles are common in neurodegenerative disorders. Pathophysiologic mechanisms that underlie disruption of circadian rhythmicity in Alzheimer disease (AD) have been well established. Circadian biology of other neurodegenerative conditions such as Parkinson disease (PD) and Huntington disease (HD) has not been systematically studied. Current understanding of the function of the circadian system in common neurodegenerative disorders (AD, PD, and HD) is summarized later.

CIRCADIAN RHYTHMS IN PARKINSON DISEASE

PD is the second most common neurodegenerative disorder after AD. Estimated prevalence of PD is more than 1 million in the United States.[49,50] The prevalence of PD is likely to double over the next few decades.[50] Motor hallmarks of PD (tremor, bradykinesia, and rigidity) result from progressive loss of dopaminergic neurons and their projections with the nigrostriatal system. Neuronal cell loss and alteration of neurotransmission outside the basal ganglia loop contribute to development of nonmotor manifestations of PD. These manifestations include disrupted sleep/wake cycles, autonomic dysfunction, cognitive decline, and alterations in mood. Both motor and nonmotor manifestations of PD show strong diurnal oscillations. These clinical observations coupled with current understanding of progression of the neurodegenerative process of PD raise the question of whether PD is affected by chronobiology (**Fig. 1**).

Diurnal Rhythms of Clinical Features in Parkinson Disease

Examples of profound diurnal fluctuations in PD include oscillations in daily motor activity,[51–54] autonomic function,[55–60] rest-activity behaviors, and visual performance, as well as fluctuating responsiveness to dopaminergic treatments for PD. It is plausible that these fluctuations may reflect modifications in the circadian system in PD.

Actigraphy studies in patients with PD show lower peak activity levels and lower amplitude of the rest-activity cycle compared with healthy older adults.[53,54,61] Increased levels of physical activity and shorter periods of immobility during the night result in an almost flat diurnal pattern of motor activity in PD.[62,63] A fragmented pattern of activity with transitions from high-activity to low-activity periods leads to less predictable rest-activity rhythm in

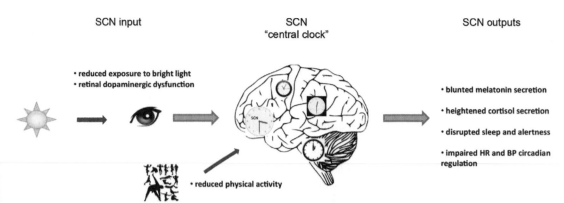

SCN input

SCN
"central clock"

SCN outputs

• reduced exposure to bright light
• retinal dopaminergic dysfunction

• blunted melatonin secretion

• heightened cortisol secretion

• disrupted sleep and alertness

• impaired HR and BP circadian regulation

• reduced physical activity

Fig. 1. A simplified scheme of the circadian system with potential causes and consequences of circadian disruption in Parkinson disease (PD). The environmental photic (light) and nonphotic (physical activity) *zeitgebers* synchronize the central circadian pacemaker (SCN) to daily light-dark and social rhythms. The SCN synchronizes other central and peripheral clocks via neuronal and humoral efferents. This internal synchronization is important for optimal physiologic function and behavior.

PD.[61] The circadian pattern of motor symptoms in PD is characterized by worsening of motor functioning in the afternoon and evening, present in both stable patients and patients with motor fluctuations.[51,64] This daily pattern occurs independently of the timing of dopaminergic medications, and may be related to circadian regulation of dopaminergic systems. Furthermore, responsiveness of PD motor symptoms to dopaminergic treatments declines throughout the day, despite the absence of significant changes in levodopa pharmacokinetics.[51,65] Nonmotor manifestations of PD, such as neuropsychiatric symptoms of PD, seem to be independently associated with reduced interdaily stability of the rest-activity cycle.[61]

Autonomic dysfunction is an important and common component of PD. Alterations in the circadian regulation of the autonomic system have been reported in PD. BP monitoring in PD shows reversal of the circadian rhythm of BP, increased diurnal BP variability, postprandial hypotension, and a high nocturnal BP load.[57,66–68] This finding is associated with a decrease of daily sympathetic activity with a loss of the circadian HR variability and a disappearance of the sympathetic morning peak.[56] Although these abnormalities are more prominent in advanced PD, suppressed 24-hour HR variability remains present in untreated patients with early PD as well[69] The prognostic significance and pathophysiologic mechanisms leading to suppressed circadian HR variability in PD remain to be determined. Although observed abnormalities arise from the peripheral autonomic ganglia, the influence of central networks such as the hypothalamus, which remains affected by neurodegenerative process of PD, may be significant.[70–72] Impairments of several sensory systems, such as olfaction and visual functions, are also reported in PD.

Similarly to motor performance, circadian fluctuations of visual performance, measured by contrast sensitivity, have been reported in PD.[73]

Impaired sleep and alertness are among the most common nonmotor manifestations of PD, and affect up to 90% of patients with PD.[74–76] Sleep maintenance insomnia is the most common sleep disorder in this population (**Fig. 2**). Other sleep disorders include sleep disordered breathing, parasomnias, and periodic limb movements disorder. Although sleep disturbances in PD worsen with progression of the disease, objective measures of sleep quality show alterations in sleep-wake cycles in patients with de novo PD.[77] The causes of sleep/wake disturbances in PD encompass the influence of motor symptoms on sleep and alertness, adverse effects of antiparkinsonian medications, and primary neurodegeneration of central sleep regulatory areas.[78–84] The role of circadian dysfunction has just recently started to be a focus of clinical studies in PD.

Markers of Circadian System in Parkinson Disease

Several studies examined markers of the circadian system in the PD population. Initial studies that focused on the secretion of melatonin reported phase advance of melatonin rhythm.[85–87] Plasma cortisol rhythms in these studies did not differ between the PD group and controls. In another study of 12 patients with PD, 24-hour mean cortisol production rate was significantly higher and the mean secretory cortisol curve was flatter, leading to significantly reduced diurnal variation in the PD group relative to controls.[88] These studies did not control for exogenous factors that are known to influence endogenous circadian rhythms, such as

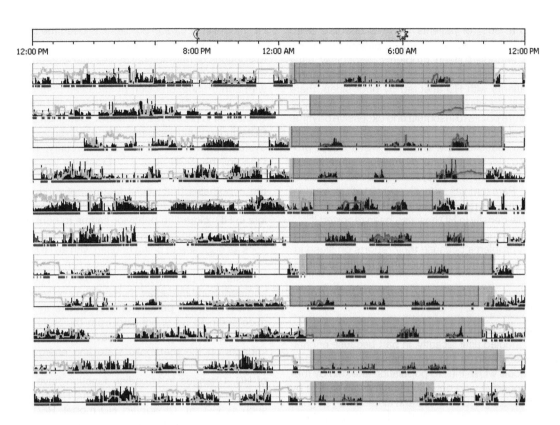

Fig. 2. Representative actigraphy record of a patient with Parkinson disease and associated sleep fragmentation and excessive daytime sleepiness. The intervals marked in blue represent sleep periods as indicated on the patient's sleep diaries.

light exposure, timing of meals, ambient temperature, and physical activity, and coexistent depression. Recent circadian investigations eliminated these methodological limitations. Using salivary dim-light melatonin onset in 29 patients with PD and 27 healthy controls, Bolitho and colleagues[89] showed a prolongation of the phase angle of melatonin rhythm in the medicated patients with PD compared with the unmedicated PD group and controls. Two other recent studies did not show alterations in the circadian phase of melatonin secretion.[90,91] However, both studies reported decreased amplitudes of melatonin secretion. Further, compared with patients with PD without excessive daytime sleepiness, patients with excessive sleepiness had significantly lower amplitudes and 24-hour melatonin area under the curve.

Temperature, perhaps the most valid marker of endogenous circadian system, was also examined in the PD population. Although 24-hour rhythms of core body temperature remain similar in PD relative to healthy controls,[92] basal body temperature is significantly lower in parkinsonian patients.[93] Patients with PD with coexistent depression have altered circadian rhythms of rectal temperature and lower amplitudes of core body temperature.[94]

Data on molecular circadian clock mechanisms in patients with PD are scarce. Time-related variations in the expression of circadian clock genes have recently been reported in patients with PD.[95] Expression levels of the clock gene Bmal1 but not those of Per1 are dampened in total leukocytes of patients with PD and correlate positively with PD severity.[95] Another study conducted in a cohort of patients with PD with early disease reported flattened expression rhythm of a major core clock gene, Bmal1.[91]

CIRCADIAN RHYTHMS IN HUNTINGTON DISEASE

HD is a neurodegenerative movement disorder caused by an abnormal trinucleotide CAG expansion in the huntingtin (HTT) gene. HD affects approximately 14 to 16 individuals per 100,000.[96] This progressive disorder is characterized by abnormal involuntary movements, cognitive decline, and behavioral/psychiatric dysfunction. Aside from these cardinal manifestations of the disease, impaired sleep and alertness are also common in the HD population.

Up to 90% of patients with HD endorse sleep problems.[97] In a cohort of 292 patients with HD, 87% endorsed sleep problems, especially early morning awakening.[98] Despite these high numbers of patients with HD affected by poor sleep, there are few studies dedicated to sleep in HD. Available literature points to insomnia and excessive daytime somnolence. Few polysomnography studies reported reduced REM and slow wave sleep, prolonged sleep onset latency, sleep fragmentation, reduced sleep efficiency, and reduced total sleep time. Parasomnias and sleep-related movement disorders are rarely present in HD. Increased sleep spindle density in HD has also been reported.[99,100] It seems that patients with HD may not recognize sleep problems because their reports on sleep instruments do not differ much from healthy controls.

Markers of Circadian System in Huntington Disease

Circadian rhythms in HD have not been systematically studied until recently, in part because of challenges related to the implementation of circadian protocols within the HD population affected by motor, cognitive, and behavioral deficits as well as by lack of recognition of sleep and circadian dysregulation in this disorder. Circadian disruption in HD has neuroanatomic correlates, because postmortem studies documented reduced expression of vasoactive intestinal peptide and arginine vasopressin, which are characteristic peptides in the SCN.[101] Actigraphy studies in patients with HD reveal a decreased level of daytime activity and increased overnight activity, leading to abnormal night/day activity ratios. Delayed sleep phase and increased REM latency have been reported in patients with HD.[102] Phase delay seems to be present in both premanifest HD mutation carriers and patients with HD.[97] Later wake-up times correlate with more prominent depressive symptoms, lower functional scores, worse and cognitive performance. Changes in melatonin secretion were also reported.[102] Dimlight melatonin onset is variable in patients with HD compared with controls. Moreover, concentrations of melatonin in serum are significantly decreased in patients with HD, with manifest patients showing more significant reductions compared with premanifest HD mutation carriers.[103] Alterations in cortisol and adrenocorticotropic hormone have been found in HD.

Circadian Homeostasis in Animal Models of Huntington disease

Informative observations on circadian function in HD have emerged in recent years from animal models of the disease. The most commonly used HD model in circadian studies has been the transgenic R6/2 mice model. R6/2 mice show profound disruptions of rest-activity cycles that worsen with disease progression.[104] This disruption is coupled with abnormal expression of circadian core clock genes in the SCN and several other brain regions. Of interest is preserved molecular regulation of the SCN during in vitro experiments, which suggests a dysfunction within the circadian circuitry, rather than in the SCN itself.[105] Emerging evidence from a transgenic sheep model of HD supports the hypothesis that social factors/networks may influence circadian rest/activity cycles and behaviors in HD; circadian behavior seems to normalize when HD sheep are kept with the normal sheep flock as opposed to being housed with an HD flock only, in which circumstances circadian disruption persists.[106] Internal desynchrony between central and peripheral circadian rhythms may be relevant to HD, because peripheral liver clocks in R6/2 mice seem to be uncoupled from the SCN control.[107] This desynchrony may have negative impacts on the metabolic state and energy homeostasis, which in turn may affect the biology of HD. Changes in circadian function have also been reported in several other animal HD models, such as HD rat, Drosophila HD model, R6/1 HD mice, and bacterial artificial chromosome (BAC) mouse model of HD.[108–110]

CIRCADIAN RHYTHMS IN ALZHEIMER DISEASE

AD is the most common form of neurodegenerative dementia and affects 1 in 9 people greater than or equal to 65 years old.[111] This disease is one of the tauopathies and its pathologic hallmark is the accumulation of amyloid-β (Aβ) and tau proteins. Sleep and circadian disruption are common in AD, affecting up to 40% of patients with mild to moderate dementia.[112] Disruption of the rest-activity cycles may be predictive of cognitive impairment/dementia. A large epidemiologic study showed increased risk of developing AD in the setting of fragmented sleep, and others reported associations between impaired cognition and poor sleep quality, low sleep efficiency, and frequent daytime napping.[113–116]

Circadian Disruption in Alzheimer Disease: Pathophysiology

Circadian dysregulation has a major impact on quality of life and represents a major reason for the institutionalization among the AD population.[117] Pathophysiologic mechanisms that underlie disruption of circadian rhythmicity in AD have been well established. Neuronal cell loss within the SCN and loss of pineal gland function are the main contributors to disrupted circadian rhythm in the AD population.[118,119] Atrophy of the SCN is associated with reduced numbers of neurons with melatonin receptors and presence of the neurofibrillary tangles.[119,120] Further, neurons that express peptide-defining SCN compartments such as intestinal polypeptide and neurotensin are also depleted in AD.[121,122] These neurochemical and neuropathologic changes within the SCN become more prominent with the progression of AD. Lack of zeitgebers necessary for the entrainment of the circadian system and coexistence of primary sleep disorders such as sleep disordered breathing are additional causes of circadian and sleep disruption in PD.

Markers of Circadian System in Alzheimer Disease

Although the changes in circadian markers in AD mimic those observed in aging, the magnitude of these changes is enhanced in AD. Circadian rhythm of temperature shows phase delay and dampened amplitude. The age-related decline of melatonin levels is more pronounced in AD relative to healthy peers.[39,123] Cerebrospinal fluid (CSF) melatonin levels are reduced in preclinical stages, and they continue to decrease with the progression of AD.[118,124,125] Alterations in amplitude and timing of cortisol and core body temperature are altered in AD as well.[126,127] There is a positive correlation between circadian rhythm disturbances and the degree of dementia in AD.[104,128,129] The amplitude of the rest-activity cycle is low in patients with AD and circadian phase becomes progressively delayed throughout the course of the disease.[130] Further, sleep duration is reduced and fragmented, and daytime becomes interspersed with frequent napping. Sleep interruption and naps during the daytime alter rest-activity rhythms, leading to a reversal of the normal rest-activity pattern, which is well documented in actigraphy studies conducted in the AD population.[129,131] Most prominent disruptions in rest-activity cycles are evident in institutionalized patients with AD.

Sleep and Circadian Function–Alzheimer Disease: Bidirectional Relationship?

The role of AD-specific neurodegeneration in the genesis of circadian disruption has been well supported in animal and human studies. However, emerging literature points to a likely bidirectional relationship between AD and circadian dysregulation.[132] Studies that used animal models of AD, including a transgenic APP/PS1 mouse model and the PLB1 triple knock-in model, have shed additional light on these associations.[133–135] The

sleep-wake states influence amyloid dynamics, and there is well-established Aβ rhythmicity in CSF.[133,136] Sleep deprivation promotes Aβ deposition into insoluble amyloid plaques, and therefore likely has a negative impact on cognitive decline.[137] Further, poor sleep quality, and specifically reduced slow wave sleep, results in neuronal hyperexcitability during sleep, which is another mechanism that promotes greater release of Aβ.[138] Similarly, sleep deprivation leads to increased Aβ levels in healthy individuals and to markedly increased Aβ accumulation in AD.[139] Cognitively intact individuals who have evidence of amyloid plaques have worse quality of sleep and sleep efficiency, and more overnight awakenings compared with healthy controls.[140]

Several circadian-based interventions have been attempted to improve sleep-wake cycles and circadian function in AD. Melatonin seems not be effective at restoring rest-activity cycles in AD, as measured by actigraphy.[135,141] Light therapy may be effective in restoring circadian rest-activity behaviors and also in improving sleep quality in the AD population.[142–144]

SUMMARY

Numerous studies have shown the importance of healthy circadian rhythmicity in maintaining neurologic homeostasis. Future research on the chronobiology of neurologic diseases will involve greater understanding of the role that circadian phenomena play at the cellular and molecular levels in the pathogenesis of brain disorders. This understanding will form the foundation for the development of new circadian-based interventions to improve clinical management of brain disorders. For example, with increasing understanding of the importance of circadian rhythmicity for brain health, one important direction will be to focus on the importance of chronopharmacology in neurologic disorders. Already considered in other medical disciplines, time of day needs to be accounted for when considering side effects and also efficacy of pharmacologic therapies for neurologic disorders. The circadian system has therefore become a novel diagnostic and therapeutic target for neurologic disorders.

REFERENCES

1. Palma JA, Urrestarazu E, Iriarte J. Sleep loss as risk factor for neurologic disorders: a review. Sleep Med 2013;14(3):229–36.
2. Culebras A. Sleep, stroke and poststroke. Neurol Clin 2012;30(4):1275–84.

3. Wang Z, Wang L, Zhang L, et al. Circadian relations among cardiovascular variables of young adults. Chronobiologia 1992;19(3–4):111–20.

4. Shimamura T, Nakajima M, Iwasaki T, et al. Analysis of circadian blood pressure rhythm and target-organ damage in stroke-prone spontaneously hypertensive rats. J Hypertens 1999;17(2):211–20.

5. Wouters A, Lemmens R, Dupont P, et al. Wake-up stroke and stroke of unknown onset: a critical review. Front Neurol 2014;5:153.

6. Elliott WJ. Circadian variation in the timing of stroke onset: a meta-analysis. Stroke 1998;29(5):992–6.

7. Manfredini R, Boari B, Bressan S, et al. Influence of circadian rhythm on mortality after myocardial infarction: data from a prospective cohort of emergency calls. Am J Emerg Med 2004;22(7):555–9.

8. Triggering and circadian variation of onset of acute cardiovascular disease. A symposium. Boston, Massachusetts, February 25, 1989 and Phoenix, Arizona, May 5-6, 1989. Proceedings. Am J Cardiol 1990;66(16):1G–70G.

9. Casetta I, Granieri E, Fallica E, et al. Patient demographic and clinical features and circadian variation in onset of ischemic stroke. Arch Neurol 2002;59(1):48–53.

10. Casetta I, Granieri E, Portaluppi F, et al. Circadian variability in hemorrhagic stroke. JAMA 2002;287(10):1266–7.

11. Gallerani M, Portaluppi F, Maida G, et al. Circadian and circannual rhythmicity in the occurrence of subarachnoid hemorrhage. Stroke 1996;27(10):1793–7.

12. Omama S, Yoshida Y, Ogawa A, et al. Differences in circadian variation of cerebral infarction, intracerebral haemorrhage and subarachnoid haemorrhage by situation at onset. J Neurol Neurosurg Psychiatry 2006;77(12):1345–9.

13. Rhoney DH, Coplin WM, Lin Y, et al. Time of day, outcome, and response to thrombolytic therapy: the National Institute of Neurological Disorders and Stroke Recombinant Tissue Plasminogen Activator Stroke Trial experience. J Stroke Cerebrovasc Dis 2010;19(1):40–8.

14. Hodoglugil U, Gunaydin B, Yardim S, et al. Seasonal variation in the effect of a fixed dose of heparin on activated clotting time in patients prepared for open-heart surgery. Chronobiol Int 2001;18(5):865–73.

15. Zhang R, Lahens NF, Ballance HI, et al. A circadian gene expression atlas in mammals: implications for biology and medicine. Proc Natl Acad Sci U S A 2014;111(45):16219–24.

16. Young ME, Razeghi P, Taegtmeyer H. Clock genes in the heart: characterization and attenuation with hypertrophy. Circ Res 2001;88(11):1142–50.

17. McNamara P, Seo SB, Rudic RD, et al. Regulation of CLOCK and MOP4 by nuclear hormone receptors in the vasculature: a humoral mechanism to reset a peripheral clock. Cell 2001;105(7):877–89.

18. Takeda N, Maemura K, Horie S, et al. Thrombomodulin is a clock-controlled gene in vascular endothelial cells. J Biol Chem 2007;282(45):32561–7.

19. Nonaka H, Emoto N, Ikeda K, et al. Angiotensin II induces circadian gene expression of clock genes in cultured vascular smooth muscle cells. Circulation 2001;104(15):1746–8.

20. Leibetseder V, Humpeler S, Svoboda M, et al. Clock genes display rhythmic expression in human hearts. Chronobiol Int 2009;26(4):621–36.

21. Yang G, Jia Z, Aoyagi T, et al. Systemic PPARgamma deletion impairs circadian rhythms of behavior and metabolism. PLoS One 2012;7(8):e38117.

22. Masuki S, Todo T, Nakano Y, et al. Reduced alpha-adrenoceptor responsiveness and enhanced baroreflex sensitivity in Cry-deficient mice lacking a biological clock. J Physiol 2005;566(Pt 1):213–24.

23. Xie Z, Su W, Liu S, et al. Smooth-muscle BMAL1 participates in blood pressure circadian rhythm regulation. J Clin Invest 2015;125(1):324–36.

24. Schroder EA, Lefta M, Zhang X, et al. The cardiomyocyte molecular clock, regulation of Scn5a, and arrhythmia susceptibility. Am J Physiol Cell Physiol 2013;304(10):C954–65.

25. Martino TA, Oudit GY, Herzenberg AM, et al. Circadian rhythm disorganization produces profound cardiovascular and renal disease in hamsters. Am J Physiol Regul Integr Comp Physiolphysiology 2008;294(5):R1675–83.

26. Mohri T, Emoto N, Nonaka H, et al. Alterations of circadian expressions of clock genes in Dahl salt-sensitive rats fed a high-salt diet. Hypertension 2003;42(2):189–94.

27. Durgan DJ, Hotze MA, Tomlin TM, et al. The intrinsic circadian clock within the cardiomyocyte. Am J Physiol Heart Circ Physiol 2005;289(4):H1530–41.

28. Tischkau SA, Barnes JA, Lin FJ, et al. Oscillation and light induction of timeless mRNA in the mammalian circadian clock. J Neurosci 1999;19(12):RC15.

29. Karmarkar SW, Bottum KM, Krager SL, et al. ERK/MAPK is essential for endogenous neuroprotection in SCN2.2 cells. PLoS One 2011;6(8):e23493.

30. Drug therapy for Parkinson's disease. Med Lett Drugs Ther 1975;17(8):33–4.

31. Czeisler CA, Dumont M, Duffy JF, et al. Association of sleep-wake habits in older people with changes in output of circadian pacemaker. Lancet 1992;340(8825):933–6.

32. Duffy JF, Zeitzer JM, Rimmer DW, et al. Peak of circadian melatonin rhythm occurs later within the sleep of older subjects. Am J Physiol Endocrinol Metab 2002;282(2):E297–303.

33. Hofman MA. The human circadian clock and aging. Chronobiol Int 2000;17(3):245–59.

34. Touitou Y, Haus E. Alterations with aging of the endocrine and neuroendocrine circadian system in humans. Chronobiol Int 2000;17(3):369–90.

35. Turek FW, Penev P, Zhang Y, et al. Effects of age on the circadian system. Neurosci Biobehav Rev 1995;19(1):53–8.

36. van Coevorden A, Mockel J, Laurent E, et al. Neuroendocrine rhythms and sleep in aging men. Am J Physiol 1991;260(4 Pt 1):E651–61.

37. Harper DG, Volicer L, Stopa EG, et al. Disturbance of endogenous circadian rhythm in aging and Alzheimer disease. Am J Geriatr Psychiatry 2005; 13(5):359–68.

38. Carrier J, Paquet J, Morettini J, et al. Phase advance of sleep and temperature circadian rhythms in the middle years of life in humans. Neurosci Lett 2002;320(1–2):1–4.

39. Wu YH, Swaab DF. The human pineal gland and melatonin in aging and Alzheimer's disease. J Pineal Res 2005;38(3):145–52.

40. Sharma M, Palacios-Bois J, Schwartz G, et al. Circadian rhythms of melatonin and cortisol in aging. Biol Psychiatry 1989;25(3):305–19.

41. Van Cauter E, Leproult R, Kupfer DJ. Effects of gender and age on the levels and circadian rhythmicity of plasma cortisol. J Clin Endocrinol Metab 1996;81(7):2468–73.

42. Born J, Spath-Schwalbe E, Schwakenhofer H, et al. Influences of corticotropin-releasing hormone, adrenocorticotropin, and cortisol on sleep in normal man. J Clin Endocrinol Metab 1989;68(5):904–11.

43. Dallman MF, Strack AM, Akana SF, et al. Feast and famine: critical role of glucocorticoids with insulin in daily energy flow. Front Neuroendocrinol 1993; 14(4):303–47.

44. Ferrari E, Arcaini A, Gornati R, et al. Pineal and pituitary-adrenocortical function in physiological aging and in senile dementia. Exp Gerontol 2000; 35(9–10):1239–50.

45. Magri F, Locatelli M, Balza G, et al. Changes in endocrine circadian rhythms as markers of physiological and pathological brain aging. Chronobiol Int 1997;14(4):385–96.

46. Kawinska A, Dumont M, Selmaoui B, et al. Are modifications of melatonin circadian rhythm in the middle years of life related to habitual patterns of light exposure? J Biol Rhythms 2005; 20(5):451–60.

47. Zeitzer JM, Daniels JE, Duffy JF, et al. Do plasma melatonin concentrations decline with age? Am J Med 1999;107(5):432–6.

48. Zeitzer JM, Duffy JF, Lockley SW, et al. Plasma melatonin rhythms in young and older humans during sleep, sleep deprivation, and wake. Sleep 2007;30(11):1437–43.

49. Alves G, Forsaa EB, Pedersen KF, et al. Epidemiology of Parkinson's disease. J Neurol 2008; 255(Suppl 5):18–32.

50. Dorsey ER, Constantinescu R, Thompson JP, et al. Projected number of people with Parkinson disease in the most populous nations, 2005 through 2030. Neurology 2007;68(5):384–6.

51. Bonuccelli U, Del Dotto P, Lucetti C, et al. Diurnal motor variations to repeated doses of levodopa in Parkinson's disease. Clin Neuropharmacol 2000; 23(1):28–33.

52. Nutt JG, Woodward WR, Carter JH, et al. Influence of fluctuations of plasma large neutral amino acids with normal diets on the clinical response to levodopa. J Neurol Neurosurg Psychiatry 1989;52(4): 481–7.

53. van Hilten JJ, Kabel JF, Middelkoop HA, et al. Assessment of response fluctuations in Parkinson's disease by ambulatory wrist activity monitoring. Acta Neurol Scand 1993;87(3):171–7.

54. van Hilten JJ, Middelkoop HA, Kerkhof GA, et al. A new approach in the assessment of motor activity in Parkinson's disease. J Neurol Neurosurg Psychiatry 1991;54(11):976–9.

55. Arias-Vera JR, Mansoor GA, White WB. Abnormalities in blood pressure regulation in a patient with Parkinson's disease. Am J Hypertens 2003;16(7): 612–3.

56. Devos D, Kroumova M, Bordet R, et al. Heart rate variability and Parkinson's disease severity. J Neural Transm 2003;110(9):997–1011.

57. Ejaz AA, Sekhon IS, Munjal S. Characteristic findings on 24-h ambulatory blood pressure monitoring in a series of patients with Parkinson's disease. Eur J Intern Med 2006;17(6):417–20.

58. Mihci E, Kardelen F, Dora B, et al. Orthostatic heart rate variability analysis in idiopathic Parkinson's disease. Acta Neurol Scand 2006;113(5):288–93.

59. Pathak A, Senard JM. Blood pressure disorders during Parkinson's disease: epidemiology, pathophysiology and management. Expert Rev Neurother 2006;6(8):1173–80.

60. Pursiainen V, Haapaniemi TH, Korpelainen JT, et al. Circadian heart rate variability in Parkinson's disease. J Neurol 2002;249(11):1535–40.

61. Whitehead DL, Davies AD, Playfer JR, et al. Circadian rest-activity rhythm is altered in Parkinson's disease patients with hallucinations. Mov Disord 2008;23(8):1137–45.

62. van Hilten B, Hoff JI, Middelkoop HA, et al. Sleep disruption in Parkinson's disease. Assessment by continuous activity monitoring. Arch Neurol 1994; 51(9):922–8.

63. van Hilten JJ, Hoogland G, van der Velde EA, et al. Diurnal effects of motor activity and fatigue in Parkinson's disease. J Neurol Neurosurg Psychiatry 1993;56(8):874–7.

64. Piccini P, Del Dotto P, Pardini C, et al. Diurnal worsening in Parkinson patients treated with levodopa. Riv Neurol 1991;61(6):219–24 [in Italian].

65. Nyholm D, Lennernas H, Johansson A, et al. Circadian rhythmicity in levodopa pharmacokinetics in patients with Parkinson disease. Clin Neuropharmacol 2010;33(4):181–5.

66. Kallio M, Haapaniemi T, Turkka J, et al. Heart rate variability in patients with untreated Parkinson's disease. Eur J Neurol 2000;7(6):667–72.

67. Plaschke M, Trenkwalder P, Dahlheim H, et al. Twenty-four-hour blood pressure profile and blood pressure responses to head-up tilt tests in Parkinson's disease and multiple system atrophy. J Hypertens 1998;16(10):1433–41.

68. Senard JM, Chamontin B, Rascol A, et al. Ambulatory blood pressure in patients with Parkinson's disease without and with orthostatic hypotension. Clin Auton Res 1992;2(2):99–104.

69. Haapaniemi TH, Pursiainen V, Korpelainen JT, et al. Ambulatory ECG and analysis of heart rate variability in Parkinson's disease. J Neurol Neurosurg Psychiatry 2001;70(3):305–10.

70. Mochizuki A, Komatsuzaki Y, Shoji S. Association of Lewy bodies and glial cytoplasmic inclusions in the brain of Parkinson's disease. Acta Neuropathol 2002;104(5):534–7.

71. Wakabayashi K, Takahashi H. Neuropathology of autonomic nervous system in Parkinson's disease. Eur Neurol 1997;38(Suppl 2):2–7.

72. Langston J. The hypothalamus in Parkinson's disease. Ann Neurol 1978;3:129–33.

73. Struck LK, Rodnitzky RL, Dobson JK. Circadian fluctuations of contrast sensitivity in Parkinson's disease. Neurology 1990;40(3 Pt 1):467–70.

74. Factor SA, McAlarney T, Sanchez-Ramos JR, et al. Sleep disorders and sleep effect in Parkinson's disease. Mov Disord 1990;5(4):280–5.

75. Lees AJ, Blackburn NA, Campbell VL. The nighttime problems of Parkinson's disease. Clin Neuropharmacol 1988;11(6):512–9.

76. Tandberg E, Larsen JP, Karlsen K. A community-based study of sleep disorders in patients with Parkinson's disease. Mov Disord 1998;13(6):895–9.

77. Placidi F, Izzi F, Romigi A, et al. Sleep-wake cycle and effects of cabergoline monotherapy in de novo Parkinson's disease patients. An ambulatory polysomnographic study. J Neurol 2008;255(7):1032–7.

78. Fabbrini G, Barbanti P, Aurilia C, et al. Excessive daytime somnolence in Parkinson's disease. Follow-up after 1 year of treatment. Neurol Sci 2003;24(3):178–9.

79. Fabbrini G, Barbanti P, Aurilia C, et al. Excessive daytime sleepiness in de novo and treated Parkinson's disease. Mov Disord 2002;17(5):1026–30.

80. Fronczek R, Overeem S, Lee SY, et al. Hypocretin (orexin) loss in Parkinson's disease. Brain 2007;130(Pt 6):1577–85.

81. Linazasoro G, Marti Masso JF, Suarez JA. Nocturnal akathisia in Parkinson's disease: treatment with clozapine. Mov Disord 1993;8(2):171–4.

82. Rye DB. Sleepiness and unintended sleep in Parkinson's disease. Curr Treat Options Neurol 2003;5(3):231–9.

83. Rye DB, Bliwise DL, Dihenia B, et al. FAST TRACK: daytime sleepiness in Parkinson's disease. J Sleep Res 2000;9(1):63–9.

84. Stack EL, Ashburn AM. Impaired bed mobility and disordered sleep in Parkinson's disease. Mov Disord 2006;21(9):1340–2.

85. Bordet R, Devos D, Brique S, et al. Study of circadian melatonin secretion pattern at different stages of Parkinson's disease. Clin Neuropharmacol 2003;26(2):65–72.

86. Fertl E, Auff E, Doppelbauer A, et al. Circadian secretion pattern of melatonin in de novo parkinsonian patients: evidence for phase-shifting properties of l-dopa. J Neural Transm 1993;5(3):227–34.

87. Fertl E, Auff E, Doppelbauer A, et al. Circadian secretion pattern of melatonin in Parkinson's disease. J Neural Transm Park Dis Dement Sect 1991;3(1):41–7.

88. Hartmann A, Veldhuis JD, Deuschle M, et al. Twenty-four hour cortisol release profiles in patients with Alzheimer's and Parkinson's disease compared to normal controls: ultradian secretory pulsatility and diurnal variation. Neurobiol Aging 1997;18(3):285–9.

89. Bolitho SJ, Naismith SL, Rajaratnam SM, et al. Disturbances in melatonin secretion and circadian sleep-wake regulation in Parkinson disease. Sleep Med 2014;15(3):342–7.

90. Videnovic A, Noble C, Reid KJ, et al. Circadian melatonin rhythm and excessive daytime sleepiness in Parkinson disease. JAMA Neurol 2014;71(4):463–9.

91. Breen DP, Vuono R, Nawarathna U, et al. Sleep and circadian rhythm regulation in early Parkinson disease. JAMA Neurol 2014;71(5):589–95.

92. Pierangeli G, Provini F, Maltoni P, et al. Nocturnal body core temperature falls in Parkinson's disease but not in Multiple-System Atrophy. Mov Disord 2001;16(2):226–32.

93. Cagnacci A, Bonuccelli U, Melis GB, et al. Effect of naloxone on body temperature in postmenopausal women with Parkinson's disease. Life Sci 1990;46(17):1241–7.

94. Suzuki K, Miyamoto T, Miyamoto M, et al. Circadian variation of core body temperature in Parkinson disease patients with depression: a potential biological marker for depression in Parkinson disease. Neuropsychobiology 2007;56(4):172–9.

95. Cai Y, Liu S, Sothern RB, et al. Expression of clock genes Per1 and Bmal1 in total leukocytes in health and Parkinson's disease. Eur J Neurol 2010;17(4): 550–4.

96. Morrison PJ. Accurate prevalence and uptake of testing for Huntington's disease. Lancet Neurol 2010;9(12):1147.

97. Goodman AO, Morton AJ, Barker RA. Identifying sleep disturbances in Huntington's disease using a simple disease-focused questionnaire. PLoS Curr 2010;2:RRN1189.

98. Taylor N, Bramble D. Sleep disturbance and Huntingdon's disease. Br J Psychiatry 1997;171:393.

99. Wiegand M, Moller AA, Lauer CJ, et al. Nocturnal sleep in Huntington's disease. J Neurol 1991; 238(4):203–8.

100. Emser W, Brenner M, Stober T, et al. Changes in nocturnal sleep in Huntington's and Parkinson's disease. J Neurol 1988;235(3):177–9.

101. van Wamelen DJ, Aziz NA, Anink JJ, et al. Suprachiasmatic nucleus neuropeptide expression in patients with Huntington's Disease. Sleep 2013;36(1): 117–25.

102. Aziz NA, Anguelova GV, Marinus J, et al. Sleep and circadian rhythm alterations correlate with depression and cognitive impairment in Huntington's disease. Parkinsonism Relat Disord 2010;16(5): 345–50.

103. Kalliolia E, Silajdzic E, Nambron R, et al. Plasma melatonin is reduced in Huntington's disease. Mov Disord 2014;29(12):1511–5.

104. Morton AJ, Wood NI, Hastings MH, et al. Disintegration of the sleep-wake cycle and circadian timing in Huntington's disease. J Neurosci 2005; 25(1):157–63.

105. Kudo T, Schroeder A, Loh DH, et al. Dysfunctions in circadian behavior and physiology in mouse models of Huntington's disease. Exp Neurol 2011; 228(1):80–90.

106. Morton AJ, Rudiger SR, Wood NI, et al. Early and progressive circadian abnormalities in Huntington's disease sheep are unmasked by social environment. Hum Mol Genet 2014;23(13):3375–83.

107. Maywood ES, Fraenkel E, McAllister CJ, et al. Disruption of peripheral circadian timekeeping in a mouse model of Huntington's disease and its restoration by temporally scheduled feeding. J Neurosci 2010;30(30):10199–204.

108. Schroeder AM, Loh DH, Jordan MC, et al. Baroreceptor reflex dysfunction in the BACHD mouse model of Huntington's disease. PLoS Curr 2011;3: RRN1266.

109. Gonzales E, Yin J. *Drosophila* models of Huntington's Disease exhibit sleep abnormalities. PLoS Curr 2010;2.

110. Bode FJ, Stephan M, Wiehager S, et al. Increased numbers of motor activity peaks during light cycle are associated with reductions in adrenergic alpha(2)-receptor levels in a transgenic Huntington's disease rat model. Behav Brain Res 2009; 205(1):175–82.

111. Cummings JL, Isaacson RS, Schmitt FA, et al. A practical algorithm for managing Alzheimer's disease: what, when, and why? Ann Clin Transl Neurol 2015;2(3):307–23.

112. Moran M, Lynch CA, Walsh C, et al. Sleep disturbance in mild to moderate Alzheimer's disease. Sleep Med 2005;6(4):347–52.

113. Yaffe K, Laffan AM, Harrison SL, et al. Sleep-disordered breathing, hypoxia, and risk of mild cognitive impairment and dementia in older women. JAMA 2011;306(6):613–9.

114. Potvin O, Lorrain D, Forget H, et al. Sleep quality and 1-year incident cognitive impairment in community-dwelling older adults. Sleep 2012; 35(4):491–9.

115. Lim AS, Kowgier M, Yu L, et al. Sleep fragmentation and the risk of incident Alzheimer's disease and cognitive decline in older persons. Sleep 2013; 36(7):1027–32.

116. Blackwell T, Yaffe K, Ancoli-Israel S, et al. Association of sleep characteristics and cognition in older community-dwelling men: the MrOS sleep study. Sleep 2011;34(10):1347–56.

117. Bianchetti A, Scuratti A, Zanetti O, et al. Predictors of mortality and institutionalization in Alzheimer disease patients 1 year after discharge from an Alzheimer dementia unit. Dementia 1995;6(2):108–12.

118. Wu YH, Feenstra MG, Zhou JN, et al. Molecular changes underlying reduced pineal melatonin levels in Alzheimer disease: alterations in preclinical and clinical stages. J Clin Endocrinol Metab 2003;88(12):5898–906.

119. Stopa EG, Volicer L, Kuo-Leblanc V, et al. Pathologic evaluation of the human suprachiasmatic nucleus in severe dementia. J Neuropathol Exp Neurol 1999;58(1):29–39.

120. Wu YH, Zhou JN, Van Heerikhuize J, et al. Decreased MT1 melatonin receptor expression in the suprachiasmatic nucleus in aging and Alzheimer's disease. Neurobiol Aging 2007;28(8): 1239–47.

121. Zhou JN, Hofman MA, Swaab DF. VIP neurons in the human SCN in relation to sex, age, and Alzheimer's disease. Neurobiol Aging 1995;16(4): 571–6.

122. Liu RY, Zhou JN, Hoogendijk WJ, et al. Decreased vasopressin gene expression in the biological clock of Alzheimer disease patients with and without depression. J Neuropathol Exp Neurol 2000;59(4):314–22.

123. Skene DJ, Swaab DF. Melatonin rhythmicity: effect of age and Alzheimer's disease. Exp Gerontol 2003;38(1–2):199–206.

124. Zhou JN, Liu RY, Kamphorst W, et al. Early neuro-pathological Alzheimer's changes in aged individuals are accompanied by decreased cerebrospinal fluid melatonin levels. J Pineal Res 2003;35(2):125–30.

125. Mishima K, Tozawa T, Satoh K, et al. Melatonin secretion rhythm disorders in patients with senile dementia of Alzheimer's type with disturbed sleep-waking. Biol Psychiatry 1999;45(4):417–21.

126. Satlin A, Volicer L, Stopa EG, et al. Circadian loco-motor activity and core-body temperature rhythms in Alzheimer's disease. Neurobiol Aging 1995; 16(5):765–71.

127. Giubilei F, Patacchioli FR, Antonini G, et al. Altered circadian cortisol secretion in Alzheimer's disease: clinical and neuroradiological aspects. J Neurosci Res 2001;66(2):262–5.

128. Pallier PN, Maywood ES, Zheng Z, et al. Pharmaco-logical imposition of sleep slows cognitive decline and reverses dysregulation of circadian gene expression in a transgenic mouse model of Hun-tington's disease. J Neurosci 2007;27(29):7869–78.

129. Witting W, Kwa IH, Eikelenboom P, et al. Alterations in the circadian rest-activity rhythm in aging and Alzheimer's disease. Biol Psychiatry 1990;27(6): 563–72.

130. Harper DG, Stopa EG, McKee AC, et al. Dementia severity and Lewy bodies affect circadian rhythms in Alzheimer disease. Neurobiol Aging 2004;25(6): 771–81.

131. van Someren EJ, Hagebeuk EE, Lijzenga C, et al. Circadian rest-activity rhythm disturbances in Alz-heimer's disease. Biol Psychiatry 1996;40(4):259–70.

132. Ju YE, Lucey BP, Holtzman DM. Sleep and Alz-heimer disease pathology–a bidirectional relation-ship. Nat Rev Neurol 2014;10(2):115–9.

133. Roh JH, Huang Y, Bero AW, et al. Disruption of the sleep-wake cycle and diurnal fluctuation of beta-amyloid in mice with Alzheimer's disease pa-thology. Sci Transl Med 2012;4(150):150ra122.

134. Platt B, Welch A, Riedel G. FDG-PET imaging, EEG and sleep phenotypes as translational biomarkers for research in Alzheimer's disease. Biochem Soc Trans 2011;39(4):874–80.

135. Duncan MJ, Smith JT, Franklin KM, et al. Effects of aging and genotype on circadian rhythms, sleep, and clock gene expression in APPxPS1 knock-in mice, a model for Alzheimer's disease. Exp Neurol 2012;236(2):249–58.

136. Huang Y, Potter R, Sigurdson W, et al. β-Amyloid dynamics in human plasma. Arch Neurol 2012; 69(12):1591–7.

137. Kang JE, Lim MM, Bateman RJ, et al. Amyloid-beta dynamics are regulated by orexin and the sleep-wake cycle. Science 2009;326(5955):1005–7.

138. Cirrito JR, Yamada KA, Finn MB, et al. Synaptic ac-tivity regulates interstitial fluid amyloid-beta levels in vivo. Neuron 2005;48(6):913–22.

139. Ooms S, Overeem S, Besse K, et al. Effect of 1 night of total sleep deprivation on cerebrospinal fluid beta-amyloid 42 in healthy middle-aged men: a randomized clinical trial. JAMA Neurol 2014;71(8):971–7.

140. Ju YE, McLeland JS, Toedebusch CD, et al. Sleep quality and preclinical Alzheimer disease. JAMA Neurol 2013;70(5):587–93.

141. Jansen SL, Forbes DA, Duncan V, et al. Melatonin for cognitive impairment. Cochrane Database Syst Rev 2006;(1):CD003802.

142. McCurry SM, Pike KC, Vitiello MV, et al. Increasing walking and bright light exposure to improve sleep in community-dwelling persons with Alzheimer's disease: results of a randomized, controlled trial. J Am Geriatr Soc 2011;59(8):1393–402.

143. Dowling GA, Mastick J, Hubbard EM, et al. Effect of timed bright light treatment for rest-activity disruption in institutionalized patients with Alz-heimer's disease. Int J Geriatr Psychiatry 2005; 20(8):738–43.

144. Ancoli-Israel S, Gehrman P, Martin JL, et al. Increased light exposure consolidates sleep and strengthens circadian rhythms in severe Alz-heimer's disease patients. Behav Sleep Med 2003;1(1):22–36.

Circadian Disruption in Psychiatric Disorders

Stephanie G. Jones, PhD*, Ruth M. Benca, MD, PhD

KEYWORDS

- Circadian • Psychiatric • Depression • Bipolar disorder • Genetics • Schizophrenia

KEY POINTS

- The circadian system is responsible for the temporal organization of physiologic function, and disruptions can have marked functional impacts.
- Psychiatric illnesses are often associated with disruptions in circadian rhythms, including alterations in sleep timing, core body temperature rhythms, and melatonin and cortisol secretion.
- Presence of circadian disruption and efficacy of chronobiological interventions raise questions regarding how these abnormalities contribute to disease onset, progression, maintenance, and response to treatment.
- Questions remain whether as to whether circadian disruption leads to mental health problems, and/or whether the underlying pathophysiology of psychiatric illness leads to dysregulation of circadian physiology.

INTRODUCTION

Nearly all psychiatric disorders present with circadian disruption, such as abnormalities in the timing of the sleep-wake cycle, core body temperature rhythms, and melatonin and cortisol secretion. The pathophysiologic significance of circadian abnormalities is a matter of debate, and is alternatively hypothesized to contribute to illness onset and progression (1) causally, as a direct result of genetic vulnerabilities in the circadian system that predispose to psychiatric illness; (2) secondarily, as a result of alterations in the timing of illness-related behavior leading to rhythm desynchronization; or (3) concomitantly, because of overlap in the molecular machinery and neural circuitry of psychiatric illness and the circadian system. In animal models of psychiatric disorders, there is evidence to suggest a causal link between circadian genes and behavioral disorders, but genetic data in humans are less compelling.

Nevertheless, the presence of circadian disruption in the clinical profile of most psychiatric illnesses as well as the efficacy of chronobiological interventions raise questions about how circadian timing abnormalities may contribute to disease onset, progression, maintenance, and response to treatment. Most psychiatric disorders involve some measure of circadian disruption; however, this article focuses primarily on evidence for circadian pathology in the pathophysiology of mood disorders and schizophrenia. Although sleep disturbances are a cardinal feature of psychiatric disorders, specific sleep abnormalities are not reviewed in detail here; a large number of excellent reviews have recently been written on this topic.[1–5]

CIRCADIAN SYSTEM: A BRIEF OVERVIEW

The circadian system is responsible for the temporal organization of virtually all aspect of physiology, including neuroendocrine function, body

Disclosure: The authors have nothing to disclose.
Department of Psychiatry, Center for Sleep Medicine and Sleep Research, University of Wisconsin-Madison, 6001 Research Park Boulevard, Madison, WI 53719, USA
* Corresponding author.
E-mail address: sgjones2@wisc.edu

Sleep Med Clin 10 (2015) 481–493
http://dx.doi.org/10.1016/j.jsmc.2015.07.004
1556-407X/15/$ – see front matter © 2015 Elsevier Inc. All rights reserved.

temperature, metabolic function, cognitive function, mood, and some aspects of the sleep-wake cycle. These rhythms are orchestrated by an endogenous master clock located in the suprachiasmatic nucleus (SCN) of the hypothalamus (**Fig. 1**). Although the circadian system maintains the endogenous period (τ) of rhythms in the absence of environmental input, without a force to entrain it to the environment, the length of this period is said to free run with a period close to, but not exactly, 24 hours. As such, the endogenous clock requires a regular resetting to ensure that the internal phase of the organism's clock is temporally aligned with that of the external world. This synchronization between the internal rhythm and the external world is achieved through exposure to a zeitgeber, or time giver. Although the light-dark cycle is the most potent zeitgeber for the SCN, other nonphotic factors, such as food availability, social interactions, and physical

activity, can also entrain the clock or reset circadian phase of peripheral oscillators.[6] The importance of synchronization between the physiology of the organism and the external environment cannot be overstated; it ensures not only that the organism does the right thing at the right time of day but it also imposes temporal order between the myriad biochemical and physiologic systems within the body. The physical and mental malaise often seen in jet lag or shift work is a consequence of a misalignment between the SCN and the external day-night cycle as well as between central and peripheral rhythms.[7,8]

Molecular Mechanisms of Clock Function

The circadian timing mechanism is fundamentally a cellular phenomenon, and the same core molecular machinery is responsible for creating and sustaining circadian rhythms in the SCN and

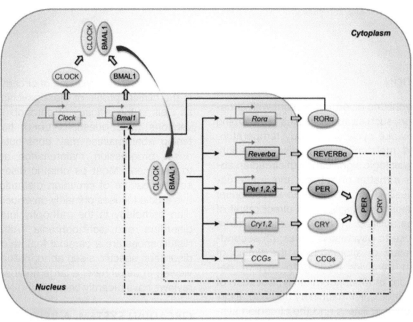

Fig. 1. Molecular machinery of the circadian clock. The core clock components CLOCK and BMAL1 heterodimerize in the cytoplasm, forming a protein complex. The heterodimer is then translocated to the nucleus and binds to E-boxes on the promoter of target genes, controlling their expression. These genes include Per1, Per2, Per3, Cry1, Cry2, Rev-erbα, Rorα, and many clock-controlled genes (CCGs). The CLOCK/BMAL1 heterodimer also stimulates transcription of Bmal1 itself, forming the positive feedback loop of the mechanism. The negative feedback loop is mainly regulated by CRY and PER, which heterodimerize in the cytoplasm, translocate to the nucleus, and inhibit CLOCK/BMAL1 transcription activity. Gene expression of Bmal1 is also regulated by REV-ERBα (inhibition) and RORα (stimulation), which compete for the same ROR elements as are present in the Bmal1 promoter. Regulation of CCG expression by the circadian clock confers rhythmicity to a variety of molecular and physiologic processes. The *straight lines* indicate stimulation and the *dashed lines* indicate inhibition. (*From* Zanquetta MM, Corrêa-Giannella ML, Monteiro MB, et al. Body weight, metabolism, and clock genes. Diabetol Metab Syndr 2010;2:53. This article is open access, distributed under the terms of the Creative Commons Attribution License (http://creativecommons.org/licenses/by/2.0), which permits unrestricted use, distribution, and reproduction in any medium, provided the original work is properly cited.)

peripheral clocks. These clocks work in a self-sustained, cell-autonomous manner, but the SCN is thought to sit at the top of this hierarchy and synchronize peripheral clocks through a wide variety of mechanisms, to be discussed later. Although this model is far from complete, some of the key clock genes in mammals include the Period genes (Per1 and Per2), the cryptochrome genes (Cry1 and Cry2), and the genes Bmal1, Rev-erbα, and Clock. At the center of this autoregulatory feedback loop are the transcriptional activators CLOCK and BMAL1, which promote the transcription of Per and Cry. The protein products of these two genes then accumulate rhythmically to repress Clock-Bmal1–driven transcription, and therefore they effectively inhibit their own transcription. CLOCK and BMAL1 also regulate their own transcription by activating the transcription of REV-ERBα and REV-ERB b. The protein products of these 2 nuclear receptors then occupy RORE DNA elements within the Bmal1 and Clock promoters. This process provides a self-sustaining oscillation that takes approximately 24 hours to complete.[9] These rhythms of clock gene expression are essential for sustaining circadian output at the level of physiology, although recent evidence suggests that the model of how individual cells keep time may ultimately prove far complex. Several questions still remain about whether cellular timekeeping in the SCN is exclusively a result of transcription-translation feedback or whether other nontranscriptional pathways, such as metabolic state, cooperate to influence circadian timekeeping at the level of the cell.[10]

Inputs and Outputs

The SCN is synchronized to the external environment by 3 major afferent pathways: the retinohypothalamic tract, the geniculohypothalamic tract, and projections from the raphe nuclei. Photic signals from the retina to neurons in the SCN lead to a postsynaptic influx of Ca^{2+}, which leads to the stimulation of the activity of cyclic AMP response element–binding protein (CREB) as well as other protein kinases. CREB initiates the transcription of the Per1 and Per2 genes. PER1 and PER2 proteins then inhibit their own expression, as well as that of the clock repressors CRY1 and CRY2, thus resetting the period of the clock. In addition to this direct input, the SCN receives photic information indirectly from the intergeniculate leaflet of the thalamus,[11–13] as well as through serotonergic input from midbrain raphe neurons. The inputs from the intergeniculate leaflet and midbrain raphe neurons are thought to provide a mechanism through which nonphotic cues, such

as feeding, exercise, and social cues, influence the SCN.[14,15]

Once entrained, output signals emerging from the SCN synchronize rhythms by sending circadian timing information to brain areas and peripheral targets involved in regulating activity, feeding, sleep-wake cycles, body temperature, and autonomic and neuroendocrine systems to optimize physiology and, ultimately, health.[16] Although not all of the mechanisms by which the SCN orchestrates these processes are clear, both axonal and neuropeptidergic signaling seem to be important. The SCN directly sets the phase relationships between itself and several brain regions via monosynaptic projections to the septum, bed nucleus of the stria terminalis, thalamus, paraventricular nucleus, and other regions of the hypothalamus. Indirectly, the SCN communicates timing in 2 other ways. First, the brain regions receiving these direct neural inputs likely communicate timing information to much of the brain through their own secondary projections. Second, the SCN can communicate circadian timing via the release of neuroendocrine factors into general circulation, either directly or secondarily.[17–19] For example, the SCN directly regulates the circadian release of corticosterone, and this hormone can be used as a timing cue in any organ or brain region that has glucocorticoid receptors. In the rodent, serotonin (5-hydroxytryptamine [5-HT]) synthesis and release within the dorsal raphe are governed by the circadian release of corticosterone, providing indirect circadian modulation of brain regions that depend on 5-HT input.[20]

EVIDENCE OF CIRCADIAN DISORDER: EVIDENCE FROM THE CLINICAL PHENOTYPE

Circadian abnormalities have long been hypothesized to a play a role in the pathophysiology of many forms of psychiatric illness. Diurnal disturbances in the sleep-wake cycle, neuroendocrine function, body temperature, and mood have frequently been described in the symptomatology of mood disorders, and, to a lesser extent schizophrenia. Moreover, for many patients, interventions that serve to stabilize or resynchronize circadian rhythms prove therapeutically effective. However, given the complex relationship between the circadian system and the sleep-wake cycle and the difficulty of accurately measuring the true phase, period, or amplitude of the circadian clock, determining whether symptoms arise from core clock abnormalities or from behaviors commonly associated with psychiatric disorders, such as improperly timed episodes of rest/activity or exposure to light, is a central challenge. In order to determine whether the circadian system is causally involved in the pathophysiology of psychiatric illness, genetic associations with clock genes are required. Although many core clock genes have been associated with either a specific psychiatric diagnosis or a dimensional feature of a disorder, most of these studies have failed to replicate in unique populations. Large, unbiased genome-wide association studies (GWAS) of psychiatric illnesses, which are able to detect the impact of common genetic variants on a phenotype, have also failed to consistently associate core circadian clock risk alleles with major depression, bipolar disorder (BPD), or schizophrenia.[21] At this point, data on circadian disruption in psychiatric illness suggests that anomalies in circadian genes may not directly cause disease, but may act to increase disease severity, accelerate disease progression, and increase the risk for poor outcomes.

Sleep and Endocrine Regulation

Major depression

Several clinical features of major depression, including diurnal mood variation, sleep abnormalities, and alterations in hormonal secretion, suggest an involvement of the circadian system. For example, dysregulation of the hypothalamic-pituitary axis (HPA) is perhaps the most frequently reported finding in patients with major depressive disorder (MDD). Although stress-related disturbances, such as increased cortisol secretion, reduced glucocorticoid receptor mRNA expression, and blunted response of the HPA axis to glucocorticoid feedback,[22] are common evidence for disturbances in the circadian regulation of the cortisol secretory profile has been mixed, and may relate to clinical severity. Some studies have reported lower morning cortisol and higher evening cortisol levels in depressed patients,[23,24] whereas others report chronically increased levels of cortisol, reflecting overactive HPA axis activity regardless of time of day, as a more common feature of depression.[25,26] Although differences in experimental processes are often offered as explanations for the discrepancies in these data, in light of the phenotypic and genetic heterogeneity of major depression, it is likely that significant circadian abnormalities, may be restricted to a subset of patients. Recent data suggests that impairments in the regulatory balance between the hypothalamus, subgenual cortex, and HPA axis may form the neural foundation for circadian dysregulation, but only in a subset of depressive patients. Decreased functional connectivity between the hypothalamus and the subgenual cortex, a region commonly reported to be dysfunctional in major depression, along with increased cortisol secretion during the circadian nadir, were shown to predict depression severity, specifically in patients with psychotic features.[27]

The pineal gland, which is responsible for the production and secretion of the hormone melatonin, is directly controlled by the SCN. As central output variable of the circadian system, a timing of melatonin output and its phase relationships with other rhythms have been widely used to characterize circadian misalignment in patients with mood disorders. Under normally entrained conditions in healthy individuals, dim-light melatonin onset (DLMO) occurs a few hours before sleep onset.[28] In women with major depression, the phase angle difference between DLMO and sleep onset has been shown to be significantly longer than in healthy subjects suggesting a delay of the internal clock, and the length of this interval was demonstrated to predict depression severity.[29] A recent report by Hasler and colleagues[30] also showed an association between circadian misalignment and depression severity in patients with MDD; although no phase angle differences were noted between the MDD and control groups, depression severity was associated with a phase angle difference between the midsleep longer period and core body temperature as well as with the angle between DLMO and core body temperature minimum, supporting a role of internal desynchrony in depressive symptoms. In addition, in subjects without a mood disorder diagnosis, a similar phase relationship was shown to predict subclinical depressed mood,[31] supporting a role for circadian misalignment in mood symptoms in both mood disorders and in healthy individuals. However, melatonin abnormalities are not a consistently reported finding in major depression, and, when present, whether they represent a primary abnormality or arise secondarily from disruptions in social and sleep rhythms is unclear. However, the possibility that internal desynchrony may play a significant role in the onset and or maintenance of mood disorders opens the door for the development of therapeutic interventions that focus on resynchronization via pathways that directly affect the clock.[32]

Bipolar disorder

A limited number of studies have assessed circadian-controlled endocrine variables in each phase of BPD to determine whether circadian disorder represents a marker of state or trait, often with divergent results.[33,34] Sleep disturbance, however, has been shown to play a consistent role in the pathophysiology of BPD during each phase of the disorder, a finding not surprising given the role of sleep in affective regulation.[35] For instance, sleep deprivation (SD) has been shown to induce hypomania or mania in a significant number of patients, and sleep disturbance is reportedly the most common prodrome of mania.[36] In euthymic patients with BPD, hypersomnia is associated with the development of future depressive symptoms.[37] Although sleep and circadian abnormalities have often been viewed as markers of the acute phases of the disorder, the presence of sleep abnormalities during remission is now well documented. A large percentage of bipolar patients report clinically significant sleep disturbance during periods of euthymia, and many meet the diagnostic criteria for insomnia.[38–41] A recent meta-analysis of actigraphy data during remission indicates that, relative to control participants, bipolar patients have longer sleep latency, sleep duration, and wakefulness after sleep onset, and lower sleep efficiency.[39] Although these findings emphasize the importance of monitoring sleep in bipolar patients, whether the described sleep disturbances represent purely circadian abnormalities is unclear. The processes of sleep and circadian rhythms are often discussed as if sleep is simply an output variable of the clock. However, although some aspects of sleep, such as rapid eye movement sleep timing, are regulated by the circadian system, other aspects are independently regulated by a distinct neural network of forebrain and brainstem sleep-promoting and wake-promoting systems.[42,43] Although these two systems engage in a significant amount of reciprocal interaction, a wealth of data supports the presence of 2 functionally and anatomically distinct systems. Assuming that sleep abnormalities are a result of circadian instability alone may obscure specific conclusions about the role of either in the pathophysiology of a given disorder. Disentangling the two processes (sleep or circadian disruption) may be particularly relevant for BPD, in which specific sleep abnormalities often change during distinct phases of the disorder, suggesting a potentially unique pathophysiological role for sleep in the maintenance of each phase.

Schizophrenia

Although the relationship between schizophrenia and circadian abnormalities has received significantly less attention than circadian dysfunction in mood disorders, several studies have documented abnormalities in both sleep cycle organization and circadian-regulated hormonal output. Commonly reported sleep abnormalities include delayed and advanced sleep onset, free-running rest-activity patterns, and irregular sleep-wake patterns. In addition, sleep architectural changes, including alterations in the timing of rapid eye movement sleep, have been reported during chronic illness as well as in the earliest stages of the disease.[44–46] Increasing evidence suggests that circadian abnormalities, particularly altered phase relationships between sleep timing and other circadian variables may play a role in the maintenance of schizophrenia, and re-aligning rhythms may improve functional outcomes. In a recent study, Wulff and colleagues[47] assessed circadian rhythms of melatonin and sleep-wake activity in a group of 20 community-dwelling patients with schizophrenia over the course of 6 weeks. To control for the impact of the lack of daily routine in this group, control subjects were selected from a group of unemployed, healthy individuals. Although all of the schizophrenic patients showed significant differences in the timing of sleep onset, offset, and midpoint relative to controls, 2 distinct profiles of sleep disruption within the schizophrenia group emerged. Sleep onset and end of the sleep period were significantly later than in controls in one-half of the group, and significantly earlier in the other. In addition, patients slept significantly longer than controls regardless of sleep onset time. Moreover, although sleep-wake onset and melatonin peaks were temporally aligned with in all subjects, in half of the schizophrenic group, these rhythms were shifted to a much later clock time, suggesting a lack of synchrony between the body's internal rhythm and the day-night cycle. Although it is conceivable that the circadian rhythm abnormality represents a primary vulnerability that drives alterations sleep-wake patterns, a more likely explanation is that the misalignment occurred secondarily to the disruption in sleep-wake and activity patterns.[47] A recent study analyzed rest-activity patterns over a 3-week period in 14 patients and reported a wide range of sleep behavior in the patient group that ranged from regular and well-entrained sleep to fragmented sleep and daytime napping.[48] Half of the patient group showed normal relative amplitudes of daytime and nighttime activity, with high-amplitude activity occurring mostly during the day and low-amplitude activity occurring at night. In contrast, the relative amplitude of the other half of the patient group was low, reflecting similar activity levels in the day and night. In contrast to the normal amplitude group, whose melatonin onset was normally aligned to the day-night cycle, in the low-amplitude group, clear melatonin onset was either impossible to detect, or, in a few cases, occurred well after habitual bedtime. Interestingly, individuals in the low-amplitude group performed significantly worse on tasks of prefrontal function relative to those patients who showed regular amplitude rest-activity cycles. Indeed, the relative amplitude of rest-activity was the most potent predictor of cognitive outcomes, suggesting that dysregulation of circadian rhythms may be associated with impaired cognitive functioning in individuals with schizophrenia. Interestingly, in a recent treatment trial of partial responders to clozapine, the addition of agomelatine, an agonist acting on both melatonin 1 and 2 receptor subtypes, was shown to improve performance on tasks of executive function,[49] suggesting that, for a subgroup of patients, circadian interventions may improve cognitive outcomes. Although intriguing, these data should be interpreted with caution, because agomelatine also exerts additional effects on the serotonergic system, and this was a small, uncontrolled pilot trial.

Evidence from the Phenotype: Gene Expression Analyses in Brain and Peripheral Tissues

Recent postmortem gene expression analyses of major depression also highlight a pathophysiologic role for disrupted circadian regulation in MDD.[50] Bunney and colleagues[50] analyzed 6 brain regions relevant to the pathophysiology of MDD, and noted a marked dampening of the circadian expression of aryl hydrocarbon receptor nuclear translocator–like (ARNTL) (BmaL1), Per2, Per3, Rev-erbα, and Per1 among other circadian regulators in subjects with MDD relative to controls. Out of the 16 cyclic genes measured, the amplitude of all was significantly decreased across all 6 brain regions in subjects with MDD, and there was also evidence for a general desynchrony of circadian oscillations between brain regions, in MDD subjects only. Moreover, circadian gene expression patterns were markedly arrhythmic, specifically in the anterior cingulate cortex (ACC), a region widely implicated in the regulation of mood. Multiple lines of evidence indicate that the ACC is disrupted in MDD, and altered circadian gene expression may play a role in symptom onset or maintenance these data provide the first direct evidence of disrupted clock brain gene expression in MDD. Although gene expression analyses, particularly in the central nervous system, support the presence of circadian gene dysregulation in mood disorders, they cannot address questions of causality. These results do, however, provide a foundation for examining how alterations of gene expression in specific brain regions may contribute to the development and progression of particular symptoms in MDD.

A recent postmortem analysis of patients with BPD and major depression reported that MT1 receptors were increased in the SCN of patients with BPD and MDD.[51] In animal models, MT1 receptor protein level in the SCN is markedly increased in response to lowered melatonin levels, and a similar compensatory mechanism may explain these increases in MT1 receptors.[52] Given that melatonin promotes sleep through its inhibitory action on the SCN via the MT1 receptor, a reduction in these receptors may play a role in the circadian profile of disrupted sleep in MDD and BPD. This reduction could also, conceivably, contribute to the efficacy of melatonin agonists on depressive symptoms.[51] Importantly, the increase in MT1 receptors was correlated with age of onset and disease duration, suggesting that the disease process, per se, may lead to circadian dysfunction rather than represent a primary abnormality.

In addition, a small number of peripheral gene expression analyses in MDD and BPD also implicate disruptions in circadian gene expression, some of which may normalize with treatment.[53,54] In one recent analysis, the rhythmic expression of Per1 and Cry1 in peripheral blood cells of depressed patients, along with the diurnal rhythmic secretion of melatonin and cortisol, failed to normalize following 8 weeks of escitalopram treatment, whereas rhythms of Per2, Bmal1, GSK-3B, and NPAS2 did normalize and were correlated with symptom improvement. Given their baseline abnormality and failure to normalize, disruptions in Per1, Cry1, melatonin, and cortisol were argued to represent trait markers of disease, whereas the dysregulation of the other gene expression rhythms were argued to arise as a consequence of disease process.[55] However, although molecular rhythms can be measured in peripheral clocks, the precise relationship between output of these cellular clocks and those in the brain are unclear, and tissue-specific factors complicate interpretation of these data.[56]

Evidence from Treatment

Another compelling piece of evidence for the role of the circadian system in mood disorders comes from the success of therapeutic interventions that affect rhythms. For example, the therapeutic efficacy of chronotherapeutic interventions such as bright light therapy, sleep deprivation (SD), and sleep phase advance have been widely shown in a variety of psychiatric phenotypes. Bright light therapy, originally intended for the treatment of seasonal affective disorder, has been shown to be effective in the treatment of nonseasonal depression, with effect sizes similar to those shown in trials of pharmacologic treatments.[57] In addition, combined with antidepressant medications, light therapy has been shown to reduce the time to symptom improvement to as little as 1 week during acute depressive episodes.[58–60] However, whether light improves mood symptoms in depression exclusively through its circadian effects is unclear. In addition to its impact on circadian phase shifting, light has broad-ranging effects on physiology and behavior, including effects on sleep, mood, alertness, and cognition, which occur independently of circadian mechanisms.[61–63]

Although the effect is transient, SD has repeatedly been shown to induce immediate symptom improvement in a broad range of depression-related phenotypes, including unipolar, bipolar, and schizoaffective depression.[64] Mood improvement occurs in approximately 40% to 60% of patients with either unipolar or bipolar depression, with relapse invariably occurring following sleep, including naps.[65] Again, the therapeutic response to SD may or may not be related to its role in remediating circadian abnormalities. SD potentiates all the monoaminergic systems that are thought to be involved in the pathophysiology of depression, most notably serotonin, and its impacts on these systems could be a component of its mechanism of action.[66] However, the role of the serotonin system in the pathophysiology of depression is not straightforward, and neither is the therapeutic efficacy of serotonergic manipulation. Only 31% of patients with MDD who participated in the Sequenced Treatment Alternative to Relieve Depression (STAR*D) project were in remission after 14 weeks of treatment with a selective serotonin reuptake inhibitor, and only 43% sustained this recovery.[67] Moreover, 5-HT depletion does not cause depression in healthy volunteers, indicating that, despite its potential role in the course of depression, serotonin imbalance is unlikely to play an exclusive role in the onset or maintenance the disorder.[68] In addition to modulating serotonin function, SD also directly influences SCN function by modifying vigilance state transitions and sleep states,[69] has been shown to modify core clock gene expression in both humans and animals.[70–72] Although the precise mechanisms through which SD exerts its therapeutic effects is complex, its modulation of circadian physiology, either directly or indirectly, likely plays a role. The benefits of sleep phase advance have also been shown effective in reducing core symptoms of depression in both BPD and MDD, although its effects are less dramatic than those associated with SD.[73] However, phase advancing the sleep cycle following a night of total SD has been shown to prevent the immediate relapse that typically occurs on the night after deprivation.[74] A few studies have also shown that all 3 therapies, bright light, SD, and sleep phase advance, termed triple chronotherapy, along with pharmacotherapy, result in a rapid reduction of depressive symptoms that endures for several weeks. For example, in 14 hospitalized, medication-resistant, depressed patients, 1 night of total SD followed by sleep phase advance(3 days) and bright light therapy (5 days) robustly improved both objective and subjective ratings of mood; this effect was observed after the SD night and mood continued to improve over the course of the intervention.[75] Similarly, a 9-week randomized trial comparing triple chronotherapy to exercise in 75 depressed patients on antidepressant therapy showed that patients in the chronotherapy group had a significantly better response relative to the exercise group. At week 9 of the intervention, 71% of the chronotherapy group versus 45% of exercise group was still responding positively to treatment.[76] A small, open-label trial also recently demonstrated that triple chronotherapy robustly improved mood and reduced acute suicidality in depressed, treatment-resistant inpatients.[77]

Interpersonal and social rhythm therapy (IPSRT), a psychosocial intervention formulated on the premise that the maintenance of rhythm stability in everyday life aids in the prevention of relapse, has also shown therapeutic promise, particularly in patients with BPD. The intervention is designed to prevent relapse by helping patients maintain medication compliance, maximize social routine regularity, and minimize the experience of stressful life events. In a randomized trial involving 175 acutely ill patients with BPD, Frank and colleagues[78] showed that patients treated with IPSRT compared with intensive clinical management experienced a longer period of stability during the maintenance phase, although there were no differences between the different therapies in the time it took to achieve clinical stability. A reduction in recurrence was also associated with higher social regularity in the IPSRT group at the end of the 2-year period. However, the specific efficacy of IPSRT versus other psychotherapy is unclear. IPSRT was one of 3 intensive psychotherapies in the Systematic Treatment Enhancement Program for BD (STEP-BD), which showed a clear role for psychotherapy in hastening recovery from depression, delaying recurrence, and maintaining stability. However, no differences were found between the 3 intensive psychosocial treatments in their therapeutic capacity.[79] A recent randomized, controlled psychotherapy trial of IPSRT versus supportive care in a group of 100 bipolar patients similarly found that, although adjuvant psychotherapy proved effective in reducing depressive and manic symptoms and social function in adolescents and young adults, the two therapies did not differ in their overall effectiveness.[80]

In addition to the success of behavioral interventions for rhythm synchronization and stabilization, nearly every antidepressant and antipsychotic medication has circadian effects, although, as with the behavioral interventions, whether these effects are related to treatment efficacy is an open question.[56] Lithium, the cornerstone of treatment of BPD, has been shown to have multiple effects on the molecular machinery of the clock. It inhibits glycogen synthase kinase 3 beta (GSK-3β) activity, which is a central regulator of NR1D1 and PER2 proteins. It also regulates early growth response 1 (ERG1), which upregulates the transcription of Per2 mRNA, ultimately leading to the transcriptional inhibition of CLOCK and BMAL1. Both in vivo and in vitro, these effects lengthen the circadian period and induce a phase delay of the clock.[81] Several candidate gene analyses have reported associations between a superior response to lithium and core clock genes, including Rev-Erbα, ARNTL, timeless (TIM), and GSK-3β, although more recent GWAS failed to replicate these findings.[82,83] Agomelatine, an MT1 and MT2 receptor agonist and serotonin 5-HT2C receptor antagonist, has shown efficacy in the treatment of major depression, and, to a lesser extent, bipolar depression, generalized anxiety disorder, and schizophrenia.[49,84–86] The compound's most potent pharmacologic properties seem to be chronobiological; along with its proven ability to phase shift human hormone release and body temperature, it has been shown to rapidly resynchronize disrupted circadian rhythms of locomotor activity and other circadian-controlled parameters.[32] Whether or not these direct chronobiological properties are primarily responsible for its clinical efficacy is unclear.

Genetic Contribution to Psychiatric Illness

Genetics of complex disorders

Although the heritability of psychiatric disorders has been consistently shown, the few genes and genetic loci identified to date account for only a small portion of the overall risk.[87,88] Both biological and phenotypic complexity, along with the limitations of current technology, serve to complicate a full genetic dissection. First, like other complex diseases, psychiatric disorders are polygenic, with each allelic polymorphism explaining only a tiny fraction of the genetic variance.

Moreover, the genetic background of the individual, including potential protective alleles along with large environmental contributions, mediates the risk of disease development or resilience. In effect, the genetic basis of a polygenic syndrome in one individual can vary significantly from that of another, and individual gene variants are neither necessary nor sufficient to cause disease. In the case of psychiatric disorders, the characterization of the phenotype may also obfuscate genetic understanding. Genetic analyses to date have focused largely on the disorder constructs outlined in the Diagnostic and Statistical Manual of Mental Disorders. Despite the clinical reliability of this system, disorder constructs do not seem to reliably group individuals with a shared cause or pathophysiology; patients with the same diagnosis often differ substantively in predominant symptom, severity, age of onset, and response to treatment. In addition, diagnostic systems are categorical, whereas complex emotional and cognitive traits are dimensional; defining the point at which normal ends and disorder begins is largely a subjective matter.[89,90] However, even in the most well-defined phenotypes, molecular and cellular-level functional changes occurring at the level of the gene are far removed from their ultimate effects on even simple traits.[91] Genes make proteins that produce cells that ultimately combine to build an extremely complex neural circuitry, sculpted by each individual's environment.[92] Even if a psychiatric phenotype is deconstructed into simpler dimensions, such as affective regulation, cognitive ability, or reward susceptibility, these constructs are far from simple; it is therefore not surprising that a single genetic variant might contribute little to even a well-characterized phenotype.

Genetic evidence from genome-wide association, linkage, and candidate gene analyses

Despite the above outlined complexities, the search for genes involved in the regulation of the circadian clock and their role in the susceptibility to psychiatric illness is an substantive research focus. Until recently, hypothesis-driven candidate gene studies have been the most common approach to elucidating genetic risk in psychiatric disorders. Notably, polymorphisms in essentially all core clock genes, including CLOCK, ARNTL1, NPAS2, GSK3β, ROR, REV-ERBα, TIMELESS, CRYs, and PERs, have been implicated in the etiology of nearly all psychiatric disorders.[93,94] Most of these studies were limited by small samples sizes and inconsistent phenotyping so results have generally been variable and difficult to replicate. However, several of these polymorphisms, including PER2, CLOCK, Gsk3β, and rev-erbα, have also been implicated in animal models of psychiatric illness, offering support for the importance of core clock genes in phenotypic features relevant to psychiatric illness. Following the publication of the human genome in 2001, and the advent of commercially produced dense single-nucleotide repeat (single-nucleotide polymorphism) arrays, GWAS (ie, unbiased genetic screening an order of magnitude larger and more detailed than previously possible) became a reality.[95] A large number of GWAS have sought to determine the relationship between psychiatric illness and circadian genes, although none has yet unequivocally identified any core clock genes with genome-wide significance; the most recent GWASs include a meta-analysis of MDD, with over 11,000 patients and controls[87]; a similarly powered study in BPD[96]; and an analysis of more than 50,000 patients with schizophrenia and matched controls.[97] Two other large GWAS, which combined 5 psychiatric disorders, and included more than 30,000 cases along with a similar number of matched controls, also failed to identify core circadian clock risk loci[21,98] (however, see also Ref.[99]). There are several reasons why these analyses would have failed to identify significant associations, in addition to the issues of phenotypic and genetic heterogeneity outlined earlier. Notably, although GWAS have the potential to provide valuable insight into the genetic architecture of complex traits, they do have significant limitations. First, GWAS are capable of detecting genetic variation modeled only by the common disease-common variant hypothesis, or the idea that susceptibility to complex disease is a function of a moderate number of common allelic variations. They cannot assess potential rare variants, including rare copy-number variants or de novo mutations, both of which have been implicated in the cause of BPD and schizophrenia.[100,101] It is also possible, given the importance of the clock to organismal fitness, that even subtle genetic anomalies have undergone significant negative selective pressure, and thus may be extremely rare in the population. In addition, epigenetic mechanisms are likely involved in the development and progression of psychiatric illness. The environment exerts potent influences on gene expression either directly or indirectly through changes in behavior, and these changes alter brain structure and function.[102]

However, although mutations in circadian genes have not been conclusively identified in GWAS, calculated risk scores in one disorder were recently shown to explain a statistically significant portion of genetic variance in another; and this effect was particularly pronounced between BPD and schizophrenia. These data suggest that, although genetic risk seems to be remarkably diffuse in all psychiatric illnesses, the portion of shared etiology between disorders is likely significant. In the recent Research Domain Criteria (RDoC) project, the National Institutes of Mental Health developed a set of guidelines to steer mental health research away from current diagnostic categories to more effectively stratify patients the goal is to begin with basic dysfunctions common to multiple disorders and to work backwards to understand the neural basis of dysfunction, rather than starting with clinical symptoms. Although not all patients with psychiatric disorders present with chronobiological abnormalities, there is sufficient evidence to suggest that a significant portion of them do, and that the stabilization of rhythms has the potential to reduce symptom severity, shorten episode severity, and limit functional impairment. Focusing research on patients for whom circadian dysregulation is a significant feature may ultimately prove fruitful for identifying disruptions in neural circuitry and/or genetic vulnerability associated with the circadian system.

SUMMARY

Multiple lines of evidence support a relationship between circadian disruption in the onset, course, and maintenance of psychiatric illness, and the study of circadian phenotypes may ultimately help to uncover pathophysiological or etiological mechanisms. However, several questions still need to be addressed. It will be important to identify the distinct effects of sleep versus circadian disruption for a given illness or disease feature. Although some aspects of sleep are regulated by the circadian system, sleep is also regulated by a distinct homeostatic process, and noncircadian features of sleep play important roles in emotion regulation; reward; cognition; and, most importantly, neural plasticity, all of which are often disrupted in psychiatric phenotypes. Although there is some evidence to suggest that circadian genes are associated with psychiatric illnesses, the specificity of these associations is unclear. Moreover, we are a long way from understanding the pathophysiological implications of potential risk genes in disorders with the phenotypic complexity of psychiatric disorders. It will also be important to distinguish the role of central versus peripheral circadian clocks, as well as specific brain clocks in the disease process; and animal models are likely to prove useful in this regard.

REFERENCES

1. Sutton EL. Psychiatric disorders and sleep issues. Med Clin North Am 2014;98:1123–43.
2. Murphy MJ, Peterson MJ. Sleep disturbances in depression. Sleep Med Clin 2015;10(1):17–23.
3. Harvey AG. Sleep and circadian rhythms in bipolar disorder: seeking synchrony, harmony, and regulation. Am J Psychiatry 2008;165:820–9.
4. Dolsen MR, Asarnow LD, Harvey AG. Insomnia as a transdiagnostic process in psychiatric disorders. Curr Psychiatry Rep 2014;16:0471.
5. Benson KL. Sleep in schizophrenia: pathology and treatment. Sleep Med Clin 2015;10(1):49–55.
6. Dibner C, Schibler U, Albrecht U. The mammalian circadian timing system: organization and coordination of central and peripheral clocks. Annu Rev Physiol 2010;72:517–49.
7. Reid KJ, Zee PC. Circadian rhythm disorders. Semin Neurol 2009;29:393–405.
8. Partch CL, Green CB, Takahashi JS. Molecular architecture of the mammalian circadian clock. Trends Cell Biol 2014;24:90–9.
9. Evans JA, Davidson AJ. Health consequences of circadian disruption in humans and animal models. Prog Mol Biol Transl Sci 2013;119:283–323.
10. Reddy AB, Rey G. Metabolic and nontranscriptional circadian clocks: eukaryotes. Annu Rev Biochem 2014;83:165–89.
11. Albers HE, Ferris CF. Neuropeptide Y: role in light-dark cycle entrainment of hamster circadian rhythms. Neurosci Lett 1984;50:163–8.
12. Biello SM, Janik D, Mrosovsky N. Neuropeptide Y and behaviorally induced phase shifts. Neuroscience 1994;62:273–9.
13. Card JP, Moore RY. Ventral lateral geniculate nucleus efferents to the rat suprachiasmatic nucleus exhibit avian pancreatic polypeptide-like immunoreactivity. J Comp Neurol 1982;206:390–6.
14. Gamble KL, Allen GC, Zhou T, et al. Gastrin-releasing peptide mediates light-like resetting of the suprachiasmatic nucleus circadian pacemaker through cAMP response element-binding protein and Per1 activation. J Neurosci 2007;27:12078–87.
15. Sheward WJ, Maywood ES, French KL, et al. Entrainment to feeding but not to light: circadian phenotype of VPAC2 receptor-null mice. J Neurosci 2007;27:4351–8.
16. Silver R, Kriegsfeld LJ. Circadian rhythms have broad implications for understanding brain and behavior. Eur J Neurosci 2014;39:1866–80.
17. Mavroudis PD, Scheff JD, Calvano SE, et al. Entrainment of peripheral clock genes by cortisol. Physiol Genomics 2012;44:607–21.
18. Maywood ES, Chesham JE, O'Brien JA, et al. A diversity of paracrine signals sustains molecular circadian cycling in suprachiasmatic nucleus circuits. Proc Natl Acad Sci U S A 2011;108:14306–11.
19. Nicolaides NC, Charmandari E, Chrousos GP, et al. Circadian endocrine rhythms: the hypothalamic-pituitary-adrenal axis and its actions. Ann N Y Acad Sci 2014;1318:71–80.
20. Malek ZS, Sage D, Pevet P, et al. Daily rhythm of tryptophan hydroxylase-2 messenger ribonucleic acid within raphe neurons is induced by corticoid daily surge and modulated by enhanced locomotor activity. Endocrinology 2007;148:5165–72.
21. Byrne EM, Heath AC, Madden PA, et al. Testing the role of circadian genes in conferring risk for psychiatric disorders. Am J Med Genet B Neuropsychiatr Genet 2014;165B:254–60.
22. Gold PW. The organization of the stress system and its dysregulation in depressive illness. Mol Psychiatry 2015;20:32–47.
23. Weinrib AZ, Sephton SE, Degeest K, et al. Diurnal cortisol dysregulation, functional disability, and depression in women with ovarian cancer. Cancer 2010;116:4410–9.
24. Cizza G, Ronsaville DS, Kleitz H, et al. Clinical subtypes of depression are associated with specific metabolic parameters and circadian endocrine profiles in women: the Power study. PLoS One 2012;7:e28912.
25. Heaney JL, Phillips AC, Carroll D. Ageing, depression, anxiety, social support and the diurnal rhythm and awakening response of salivary cortisol. Int J Psychophysiol 2010;78:201–8.
26. Vreeburg SA, Hoogendijk WJ, van Pelt J, et al. Major depressive disorder and hypothalamic-pituitary-adrenal axis activity: results from a large cohort study. Arch Gen Psychiatry 2009;66:617–26.
27. Sudheimer K, Keller J, Gomez R, et al. Decreased hypothalamic functional connectivity with subgenual cortex in psychotic major depression. Neuropsychopharmacology 2015;40:849–60.
28. Benloucif S, Burgess HJ, Klerman EB, et al. Measuring melatonin in humans. J Clin Sleep Med 2008;4:66–9.
29. Emens J, Lewy A, Kinzie JM, et al. Circadian misalignment in major depressive disorder. Psychiatry Res 2009;168:259–61.
30. Hasler BP, Buysse DJ, Kupfer DJ, et al. Phase relationships between core body temperature, melatonin, and sleep are associated with depression severity: further evidence for circadian misalignment in non-seasonal depression. Psychiatry Res 2010;178:205–7.
31. Emens JS, Yuhas K, Rough J, et al. Phase angle of entrainment in morning- and evening-types under naturalistic conditions. Chronobiol Int 2009;26:474–93.
32. MacIsaac SE, Carvalho AF, Cha DS, et al. The mechanism, efficacy, and tolerability profile of agomelatine. Expert Opin Pharmacother 2014;15:259–74.

33. Kennedy SH, Kutcher SP, Ralevski E, et al. Nocturnal melatonin and 24-hour 6-sulphatoxyme-latonin levels in various phases of bipolar affective disorder. Psychiatry Res 1996;63:219–22.

34. Novakova M, Prasko J, Latalova K, et al. The circadian system of patients with bipolar disorder differs in episodes of mania and depression. Bipolar Disord 2015;17(3):303–14.

35. Walker MP. Sleep, memory and emotion. Prog Brain Res 2010;185:49–68.

36. Soreca I. Circadian rhythms and sleep in bipolar disorder: implications for pathophysiology and treatment. Curr Opin Psychiatry 2014;27:467–71.

37. Kaplan KA, McGlinchey EL, Soehner A, et al. Hypersomnia subtypes, sleep and relapse in bipolar disorder. Psychol Med 2015;45(8):1751–63.

38. Boudebesse C, Geoffroy PA, Bellivier F, et al. Correlations between objective and subjective sleep and circadian markers in remitted patients with bipolar disorder. Chronobiol Int 2014;31:698–704.

39. Geoffroy PA, Scott J, Boudebesse C, et al. Sleep in patients with remitted bipolar disorders: a meta-analysis of actigraphy studies. Acta Psychiatr Scand 2015;131:89–99.

40. Ng TH, Chung KF, Ho FY, et al. Sleep-wake disturbance in interepisode bipolar disorder and high-risk individuals: a systematic review and meta-analysis. Sleep Med Rev 2015;20:46–58.

41. Harvey AG, Talbot LS, Gershon A. Sleep disturbance in bipolar disorder across the lifespan. Clin Psychol (New York) 2009;16:256–77.

42. Benca R, Duncan MJ, Frank E, et al. Biological rhythms, higher brain function, and behavior: gaps, opportunities, and challenges. Brain Res Rev 2009;62:57–70.

43. Schwartz JR, Roth T. Neurophysiology of sleep and wakefulness: basic science and clinical implications. Curr Neuropharmacol 2008;6:367–78.

44. Keshavan MS, Prasad KM, Montrose DM, et al. Sleep quality and architecture in quetiapine, risperidone, or never-treated schizophrenia patients. J Clin Psychopharmacol 2007;27:703–5.

45. Manoach DS, Demanuele C, Wamsley EJ, et al. Sleep spindle deficits in antipsychotic-naive early course schizophrenia and in non-psychotic first-degree relatives. Front Hum Neurosci 2014;8:762.

46. Poulin J, Daoust AM, Forest G, et al. Sleep architecture and its clinical correlates in first episode and neuroleptic-naive patients with schizophrenia. Schizophr Res 2003;62:147–53.

47. Wulff K, Dijk DJ, Middleton B, et al. Sleep and circadian rhythm disruption in schizophrenia. Br J Psychiatry 2012;200:308–16.

48. Bromundt V, Koster M, Georgiev-Kill A, et al. Sleep-wake cycles and cognitive functioning in schizophrenia. Br J Psychiatry 2011;198:269–76.

49. Bruno A, Zoccali RA, Abenavoli E, et al. Augmentation of clozapine with agomelatine in partial-responder schizophrenia: a 16-week, open-label, uncontrolled pilot study. J Clin Psychopharmacol 2014;34:491–4.

50. Bunney BG, Li JZ, Walsh DM, et al. Circadian dysregulation of clock genes: clues to rapid treatments in major depressive disorder. Mol Psychiatry 2015; 20:48–55.

51. Wu YH, Ursinus J, Zhou JN, et al. Alterations of melatonin receptors MT1 and MT2 in the hypothalamic suprachiasmatic nucleus during depression. J Affect Disord 2013;148:357–67.

52. Pevet P, Challet E. Melatonin: both master clock output and internal time-giver in the circadian clocks network. J Physiol Paris 2011;105:170–82.

53. Lavebratt C, Sjoholm LK, Soronen P, et al. CRY2 is associated with depression. PLoS One 2010;5: e9407.

54. McCarthy MJ, Wei H, Marnoy Z, et al. Genetic and clinical factors predict lithium's effects on PER2 gene expression rhythms in cells from bipolar disorder patients. Transl Psychiatry 2013;3:e318.

55. Li SX, Liu LJ, Xu LZ, et al. Diurnal alterations in circadian genes and peptides in major depressive disorder before and after escitalopram treatment. Psychoneuroendocrinology 2013;38:2789–99.

56. Zhang R, Lahens NF, Ballance HI, et al. A circadian gene expression atlas in mammals: implications for biology and medicine. Proc Natl Acad Sci U S A 2014;111:16219–24.

57. Golden RN, Gaynes BN, Ekstrom RD, et al. The efficacy of light therapy in the treatment of mood disorders: a review and meta-analysis of the evidence. Am J Psychiatry 2005;162:656–62.

58. Benedetti F, Colombo C, Pontiggia A, et al. Morning light treatment hastens the antidepressant effect of citalopram: a placebo-controlled trial. J Clin Psychiatry 2003;64:648–53.

59. Martiny K, Lunde M, Unden M, et al. Adjunctive bright light in non-seasonal major depression: results from clinician-rated depression scales. Acta Psychiatr Scand 2005;112:117–25.

60. Martiny K, Lunde M, Unden M, et al. Adjunctive bright light in non-seasonal major depression: results from patient-reported symptom and well-being scales. Acta Psychiatr Scand 2005;111: 453–9.

61. Hubbard J, Ruppert E, Gropp CM, et al. Non-circadian direct effects of light on sleep and alertness: lessons from transgenic mouse models. Sleep Med Rev 2013;17:445–52.

62. Bedrosian TA, Nelson RJ. Influence of the modern light environment on mood. Mol Psychiatry 2013; 18:751–7.

63. Bedrosian TA, Vaughn CA, Galan A, et al. Nocturnal light exposure impairs affective

responses in a wavelength-dependent manner. J Neurosci 2013;33:13081–7.

64. Benedetti F, Colombo C. Sleep deprivation in mood disorders. Neuropsychobiology 2011;64:141–51.

65. Wu JC, Bunney WE. The biological basis of an antidepressant response to sleep deprivation and relapse: review and hypothesis. Am J Psychiatry 1990;147:14–21.

66. Dallaspezia S, Benedetti F. Sleep deprivation therapy for depression. Curr Top Behav Neurosci 2015;25:483–502.

67. Nelson JC. The STAR*D study: a four-course meal that leaves us wanting more. Am J Psychiatry 2006;163:1864–6.

68. Price LH, Charney DS, Delgado PL, et al. Serotonin function and depression: neuroendocrine and mood responses to intravenous L-tryptophan in depressed patients and healthy comparison subjects. Am J Psychiatry 1991;148:1518–25.

69. Deboer T, Vansteensel MJ, Detari L, et al. Sleep states alter activity of suprachiasmatic nucleus neurons. Nat Neurosci 2003;6:1086–90.

70. Ackermann K, Plomp R, Lao O, et al. Effect of sleep deprivation on rhythms of clock gene expression and melatonin in humans. Chronobiol Int 2013;30: 901–9.

71. Archer SN, Laing EE, Moller-Levet CS, et al. Mistimed sleep disrupts circadian regulation of the human transcriptome. Proc Natl Acad Sci U S A 2014; 111:E682–91.

72. Moller-Levet CS, Archer SN, Bucca G, et al. Effects of insufficient sleep on circadian rhythmicity and expression amplitude of the human blood transcriptome. Proc Natl Acad Sci U S A 2013;110: E1132–41.

73. Souetre E, Salvati E, Pringuey D, et al. Antidepressant effects of the sleep/wake cycle phase advance. Preliminary report. J Affect Disord 1987; 12:41–6.

74. Berger M, Vollmann J, Hohagen F, et al. Sleep deprivation combined with consecutive sleep phase advance as a fast-acting therapy in depression: an open pilot trial in medicated and unmedicated patients. Am J Psychiatry 1997;154:870–2.

75. Echizenya M, Suda H, Takeshima M, et al. Total sleep deprivation followed by sleep phase advance and bright light therapy in drug-resistant mood disorders. J Affect Disord 2013;144:28–33.

76. Martiny K, Refsgaard E, Lund V, et al. A 9-week randomized trial comparing a chronotherapeutic intervention (wake and light therapy) to exercise in major depressive disorder patients treated with duloxetine. J Clin Psychiatry 2012;73: 1234–42.

77. Sahlem GL, Kalivas B, Fox JB, et al. Adjunctive triple chronotherapy (combined total sleep deprivation, sleep phase advance, and bright light

therapy) rapidly improves mood and suicidality in suicidal depressed inpatients: an open label pilot study. J Psychiatr Res 2014;59:101–7.

78. Frank E, Kupfer DJ, Thase ME, et al. Two-year outcomes for interpersonal and social rhythm therapy in individuals with bipolar I disorder. Arch Gen Psychiatry 2005;62:996–1004.

79. Miklowitz DJ, Otto MW, Frank E, et al. Psychosocial treatments for bipolar depression: a 1-year randomized trial from the systematic treatment enhancement program. Arch Gen Psychiatry 2007;64:419–26.

80. Inder ML, Crowe MT, Luty SE, et al. Randomized, controlled trial of interpersonal and social rhythm therapy for young people with bipolar disorder. Bipolar Disord 2015;17:128–38.

81. Geddes JR, Miklowitz DJ. Treatment of bipolar disorder. Lancet 2013;381:1672–82.

82. Geoffroy PA, Bellivier F, Leboyer M, et al. Can the response to mood stabilizers be predicted in bipolar disorder? Front Biosci (Elite Ed) 2014;6:120–38.

83. Rybakowski JK. Response to lithium in bipolar disorder: clinical and genetic findings. ACS Chem Neurosci 2014;5(6):413–21.

84. Fornaro M, McCarthy MJ, De Berardis D, et al. Adjunctive agomelatine therapy in the treatment of acute bipolar II depression: a preliminary open label study. Neuropsychiatr Dis Treat 2013;9:243–51.

85. Stein DJ, Ahokas A, Albarran C, et al. Agomelatine prevents relapse in generalized anxiety disorder: a 6-month randomized, double-blind, placebo-controlled discontinuation study. J Clin Psychiatry 2012;73:1002–8.

86. Stein DJ, Ahokas A, Marquez MS, et al. Agomelatine in generalized anxiety disorder: an active comparator and placebo-controlled study. J Clin Psychiatry 2014;75:362–8.

87. Ripke S, Wray NR, Lewis CM, et al. A mega-analysis of genome-wide association studies for major depressive disorder. Mol Psychiatry 2013;18: 497–511.

88. Stoltenberg SF, Burmeister M. Recent progress in psychiatric genetics–some hope but no hype. Hum Mol Genet 2000;9:927–35.

89. Casey BJ, Craddock N, Cuthbert BN, et al. DSM-5 and RDoC: progress in psychiatry research? Nat Rev Neurosci 2013;14:810–4.

90. Craddock N, Owen MJ. The Kraepelinian dichotomy - going, going... but still not gone. Br J Psychiatry 2010;196:92–5.

91. Zhao X, Yang Y, Sun BF, et al. FTO and obesity: mechanisms of association. Curr Diab Rep 2014; 14:486.

92. Albert FW, Kruglyak L. The role of regulatory variation in complex traits and disease. Nat Rev Genet 2015;16:197–212.

93. Etain B, Milhiet V, Bellivier F, et al. Genetics of circadian rhythms and mood spectrum disorders. Eur Neuropsychopharmacol 2011;21(Suppl 4):S676–82.

94. Pritchett D, Wulff K, Oliver PL, et al. Evaluating the links between schizophrenia and sleep and circadian rhythm disruption. J Neural Transm 2012; 119:1061–75.

95. Venter JC, Adams MD, Myers EW, et al. The sequence of the human genome. Science 2001; 291:1304–51.

96. Large-scale genome-wide association analysis of bipolar disorder identifies a new susceptibility locus near ODZ4. Nat Genet 2011;43:977–83.

97. Ripke S, O'Dushlaine C, Chambert K, et al. Genome-wide association analysis identifies 13 new risk loci for schizophrenia. Nat Genet 2013;45:1150–9.

98. Lee SH, Ripke S, Neale BM, et al. Genetic relationship between five psychiatric disorders estimated from genome-wide SNPs. Nat Genet 2013;45: 984–94.

99. McCarthy MJ, Nievergelt CM, Kelsoe JR, et al. A survey of genomic studies supports association of circadian clock genes with bipolar disorder spectrum illnesses and lithium response. PLoS One 2012;7:e32091.

100. Malhotra D, Sebat J. CNVs: harbingers of a rare variant revolution in psychiatric genetics. Cell 2012;148:1223–41.

101. Gershon ES, Alliey-Rodriguez N, Liu C. After GWAS: searching for genetic risk for schizophrenia and bipolar disorder. Am J Psychiatry 2011;168: 253–6.

102. Weaver IC. Integrating early life experience, gene expression, brain development, and emergent phenotypes: unraveling the thread of nature via nurture. Adv Genet 2014;86:277–307.

Non–24-Hour Sleep–Wake Rhythm Disorder in Sighted and Blind Patients

Makoto Uchiyama, MD, PhD[a], Steven W. Lockley, PhD[b,c,d],*

KEYWORDS

- Circadian rhythm sleep disorders • Non–24-hour sleep–wake rhythm disorder • Free-running type
- Nonentrained type • Hypernychthemeral syndrome • Blindness • Melatonin

KEY POINTS

- Non–24-hour sleep–wake rhythm disorder (N24SWD) is a debilitating cyclic circadian rhythm sleep disorder characterized by an inability to sleep on a 24-hour schedule.
- N24SWD is rare in sighted individuals and has multiple possible causes including behavioral, sleep-wake regulation or genetic causes.
- N24SWD is highly prevalent in totally blind individuals due to a lack of light information reaching the circadian clock.
- Optimal treatment should reset the underlying nonentrained circadian pacemaker. There are currently no approved treatments for sighted patients with N24SWD although structured light therapy and melatonin treatment hold promise.
- Tasimelteon (20 mg at a fixed clock time each day), a dual melatonin receptor agonist, was recently approved to treat N24SWD in totally blind patients.

NON–24-HOUR SLEEP–WAKE RHYTHM DISORDER (FREE-RUNNING DISORDER, NONENTRAINED DISORDER, HYPERNYCHTHEMERAL SYNDROME)

Non–24-hour sleep–wake rhythm disorder (N24SWD) is defined as a "history of insomnia, excessive daytime sleepiness, or both, which alternate with asymptomatic episodes, owing to misalignment between the light-dark cycle and the non-entrained endogenous circadian rhythm of sleep-wake propensity."[1,2] The daily light–dark cycle is the most powerful environmental time cue for synchronizing the hypothalamic circadian pacemaker to the 24-hour day. Individuals who are physically or biologically isolated from a normal 24-hour light–dark cycle exhibit a sleep–wake cycle that is different from and usually longer than 24 hours.[3,4] This non–24-hour cycle leads to progressively later or progressively earlier bedtimes and wake times. N24SWD is a rare condition in sighted individuals and is characterized by a chronic steady pattern of delays, typically of approximately 1 hour per day in spontaneous sleep-onset and wake times while living under

Updated from: Uchiyama M, Lockley SW. Non-24-hour sleep–wake syndrome in sighted and blind patients. Sleep Medicine Clinics of North America 2009;4(2):195–211.

Disclosure: See last page of article.

[a] Department of Psychiatry, Nihon University School of Medicine, Oyaguchi-Kamicho, Itabashi, Tokyo 173-8610, Japan; [b] Circadian Physiology Program, Division of Sleep and Circadian Disorders, Brigham and Women's Hospital, 221 Longwood Avenue, Boston, MA 02115, USA; [c] Department of Medicine, Harvard Medical School, Boston, MA 02115, USA; [d] School of Psychological Sciences, Monash University, Wellington Road, Melbourne, VIC 3800, Australia

* Corresponding author. Circadian Physiology Program, Division of Sleep and Circadian Disorders, Brigham and Women's Hospital, Harvard Medical School, Boston, MA 02115.

E-mail address: slockley@hms.harvard.edu

Sleep Med Clin 10 (2015) 495–516
http://dx.doi.org/10.1016/j.jsmc.2015.07.006

normal environmental conditions.[1] As most individuals are usually required to live on a 24-hour social day and maintain a regular sleep–wake schedule, the sufferer displays periodically recurring problems with sleep initiation, sleep maintenance, and rising, as the circadian cycle of wakefulness and sleep propensity moves in and out of synchrony with the fixed social sleep episode.[5] Although the disorder is generally rare in sighted people, there are a considerable number of reports[5,6]; and the disorder may be more common than previously thought in individuals in their teens and 20s.[6]

N24SWD is most common in individuals who are totally blind,[1,5,7,8] with as many as one-half of totally blind patients having this disorder. In such patients, the lack of ocular light information reaching the circadian pacemaker prevents it from entraining to the normal 24-hour light–dark cycle.[7] Consequently, the circadian pacemaker reverts to its endogenous non–24-hour period, causing a chronic, cyclic sleep–wake disorder characterized by episodes of good sleep followed by episodes of poor sleep and excessive daytime sleepiness, followed by good sleep ad infinitum. There are some differences, however, between sighted and blind subjects in the etiology and expression of this disorder. We review the clinical aspects and pathophysiology of the sighted and blind patients suffering from N24SWD.

CLINICAL CHARACTERISTICS OF NON–24-HOUR SLEEP–WAKE RHYTHM DISORDER IN SIGHTED PATIENTS

The prevalence of N24SWD in the general population has not been established, but it is presumed to be rare.[1] Systematic clinical examinations of sighted patients with N24SWD are also relatively rare, although many single case reports have been described (**Table 1**).[9–35]

Clinical Features

The basic characteristics of sighted patients having N24SWD, such as sex, age, or age at onset, remain to be elucidated.[1] Hayakawa and colleagues[6] examined 57 consecutively diagnosed patients with sighted N24SWD and found that 72% of them were men. This is comparable with previous studies listed in **Table 1**, where 85% of the patients were male. The commencement of a non–24-hour sleep–wake cycle occurred mostly when patients were in their teens or 20s (see **Table 1**). Nearly all of the patients (98%) had a history of disturbed social functioning owing to inability to regularly attend school or work and about one-quarter (28%) had psychiatric disorders.

Sleep Features

By definition, a non–24-hour sleep–wake pattern is characteristic of this disorder and is usually defined from daily sleep logs and/or wrist actigraphy collected over several consecutive weeks. Sleep duration tends to be normal to long with a mean (± standard deviation) sleep duration of 9.3 ± 1.3 hours and a median of 9.0 hours.[6] Polysomnography has typically not been performed or reported in detail in such patients because sleep structure and quality on a given single night recording depends on the phase relationship between internal biological time and sleep.[36]

Fig. 1 shows representative examples of self-reported sleep–wake records in 3 patients with N24SWD; a 26-year-old woman (see **Fig. 1**A), a 22-year-old man (see **Fig. 1**B),[6] and a 30-year-old man (see **Fig. 1**C).[8] All subjects began exhibiting symptoms in their teens and had difficulty with adjusting the school and college schedules. Clinical examinations failed to reveal any abnormalities in routine electroencephalogram, MRI, hematology and biochemistry tests. Semi-structured psychiatrics interviews revealed that case 1 had adjustment disorder and case 2 suffered from major depression (according to DSM-IV criteria). Case 3 had no axis I or III disorders. Although the sleep–wake cycle clearly has a non–24-hour pattern in all 3 cases, the behavior is not identical. Case 1 shows a relatively steadily delaying free-running sleep pattern, albeit with some minor changes in sleep duration occasionally. This pattern can only be expressed in those without strong social commitments (eg, work, school) that would prevent sleep during the daytime hours. Cases 2 and 3 show more typical patterns, although they also result in substantial social isolation. In both cases, the sleep–wake cycle does not simply have a constant non–24-hour pattern; there are at least 2 distinct components that repeat cyclically. The sleep–wake cycle shows a regular "free run" when sleep is initiated during the night or early morning, close to a normal social sleep time and when natural sunlight is not available, although most sleep episodes still start during the night (see **Fig. 1**C, *middle panel*). Once the sleep onset has delayed into the morning hours, the sleep–wake cycle becomes more disrupted and seems to delay more rapidly or have a series of delayed phase "jumps." This jump tends to occur when sleep onset approaches 8 to 10:00 AM; sleep onset occurs rarely between 10:00 and 16:00 hours (see **Fig. 1**B and C).

Such phase jumps occur in about one-half of patients (54%) with N24SWD and results in a longer observed sleep–wake period on average

Table 1
Published reports of sighted patients with non–24-hour sleep–wake syndrome

Author, Year	No.	Sex	Age at First Visit (y)	Age Onset (y)	Social Status at First Visit	Period of Sleep–Wake Cycle (h)	Premorbid Psychiatric Problems	Premorbid Sleep Disorder
Eliott et al,[16] 1970	1	M	NA	NA	NA	26	—	—
Kokkoris et al,[10] 1978	1	M	34	26	Unemployed	24.8	Schizoid personality	—
Weber et al,[11] 1980	1	M	28	24	College student	25.6	—	—
Kamgar-Parsi et al,[12] 1983	1	M	32	22	Unemployed	25.1	—	DSPS
Wollman et al,[13] 1986	1	M	26	22	Student	27.4	—	—
Sugita et al,[17] 1987	1	M	25	23	Student	25	—	—
Eastman et al,[18] 1988	1	M	26	High school	NA	25	—	—
Hoban et al,[14] 1989	1	F	40	NA	Artist	25.1	—	—
Moriya et al,[19] 1990	1	M	16	15	Student	24.5–25.0	—	—
Sasaki et al,[20] 1990	1	F	22	21	NA	NA	Bipolar affective disorder	—
Ohta et al,[21] 1991	1	M	17	15	Student	24.6	—	—
Oren & Wehr,[22] 1992	2	M	22, 28	NA	NA	NA	—	DSPS
Tagaya et al,[23] 1993	1	M	20	18	Unemployed	25.3	Schizophrenia	—
Emens et al,[24] 1994	1	M	31	22	NA	25.2	—	—
Tomoda et al,[25] 1994	1	M	18	17	Student	25	—	—
McArthur et al,[26] 1996	1	M	41	41	Computer programmer	25.1	Depression, social phobia	DSPS
Uchiyama et al,[9] 1996	1	M	30	18	Designer	27.2	—	—
Yamadera et al,[27] 1996	13	10M	23.2[a]	19.8[a]	54% students, 23% unemployed, 15% employed, 8% part-time work	NA	—	—
Nakamura et al,[28] 1997	1	M	26	NA	Student	NA	—	DSPS
Shibui et al,[29] 1998	1	M	43	41	Local government officer	25.8	—	—
Hashimoto et al,[30] 1998	1	M	26	26	Student	NA	—	—
Hayakawa et al,[31] 1998	1	M	20	16	Student	25	—	—

(continued on next page)

Table 1
(continued)

Author, Year	No.	Sex	Age at First Visit (y)	Age Onset (y)	Social Status at First Visit	Period of Sleep–Wake Cycle (h)	Premorbid Psychiatric Problems	Premorbid Sleep Disorder
Akaboshi et al,[32] 2000	1	M	5	4	Kindergarten	24.9	Mental retardation	—
Watanabe et al,[33] 2000	1	M	17	17	NA	NA	—	—
Morinobu et al,[34] 2002	1	M	22	20	NA	NA	OCD	—
Boivin et al,[35] 2003	1	F	39	32	NA	NA	—	—
Hayakawa et al,[6] 2005	57	41 M	M 26.3, F 25.8[a]	20.2[a]	35% students, 39% unemployed, 21% employed, 5% part time work	24.9[a]	28% psychiatric, 2% physical problems	26% DSPS

Abbreviations: DSPS, delayed sleep-phase syndrome; NA, not available; OCD, obsessive–compulsive disorder.
[a] Mean value.

From Hayakawa T, Uchiyama M, Kamei Y, et al. Clinical analyses of sighted patients with non-24-h sleep–wake syndrome: a study of 57 consecutively diagnosed cases. Sleep 2005;28(8):949; with permission.

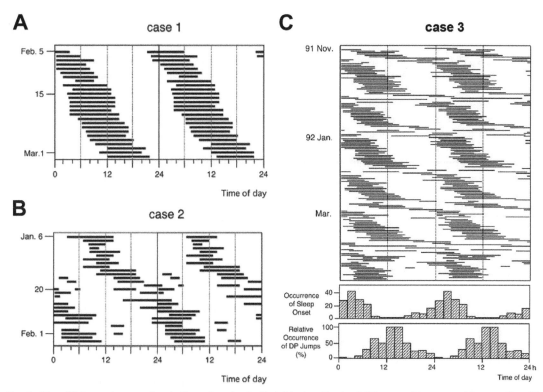

Fig. 1. Non–24-hour sleep–wake rhythm disorder in 3 sighted patients: A 26-year-old woman (*A*, case 1), a 22-year-old man (*B*, case 2), and a 30-year-old man (*C*, case 3). Sleep times (■) are double-plotted for clarity according to time of day (abscissa) and study day (ordinate). Case 1 clearly exhibits a non–24-hour sleep rhythm (24.8 hours) that remains relatively consistent. Case 2 also exhibits a non–24-hour sleep rhythm of 24.7 hours on average, although the rhythm becomes more disrupted for about a week in the middle of the data sequence. This change in rhythmicity is more clearly illustrated in case 3, who has episodes of regularly free-running sleep (24.6 hour) interspersed regularly (~every 4 weeks) with episodes where the sleep pattern delays more quickly and becomes more disrupted. These 'phase jumps' in the sleep–wake cycle are characteristic of early studies of subjects living in temporal isolation in caves and laboratory experiments, but with access to artificial light, and are most likely caused when light exposure occurs at a particular phase of the circadian cycle (see **Fig. 5** and text). Even under this nonentrained condition, the sleep onset occurs most often during the night (case 3, *middle panel*), reflecting the fact that the patient generally attempts to live on a 24-hour social day. The rapid delay in sleep–wake timing ('delay phase [DP] jumps') also occurs at a particular circadian phase (case 3, *lower panel*; see text). (Cases 1 and 2 *from* Hayakawa T, Uchiyama M, Kamei Y, et al. Clinical analyses of sighted patients with non-24-h sleep–wake syndrome: a study of 57 consecutively diagnosed cases. Sleep 2005;28:948. Case 3 *from* Uchiyama M, Okawa M, Ozaki S, et al. Delayed phase jumps of sleep onset in a patient with non-24-h sleep-wake syndrome. Sleep 1996;19:638; with permission.)

(26.1 ± 0.8 hours) than those who do not exhibit such changes (24.9 ± 0.5 hours). The nonuniform distribution of the sleep–wake behavior and the fact that sleep tends to become more abnormal when it coincides with the light phase of the day suggests that free-running sleep–wake cycle of these patients is influenced by the timing of light–dark cycle, and several experimental protocols provide support for this conclusion. Rapid changes in the phase of the sleep–wake cycle are also observed in some totally blind subjects with N24SWD, however, suggesting a potential role for nonphotic or social cues in altering sleep–wake behavior in these patients.

N24SWD and delayed sleep–wake rhythm disorder (DSWPD) may share a common pathology, and persistent sleep phase delay may increase the risk of the occurrence of N24SWD.[22,37] For example, Oren and Wehr[22] reported that 2 patients with delayed sleep-phase disorder had developed N24SWD after chronotherapy in which their sleep phase was scheduled to be delayed by 3 to 4 hours in an attempt to obtain the desired sleep phase, suggesting that, in patients with DSWPD, an enforced sleep-phase delay may trigger N24SWD. A review of previous studies (see **Table 1**) shows that persistent sleep-phase delay preceded the symptoms of N24SWD in 5 out of 39 sighted patients (13%). In a study by Hayakawa and colleagues,[6] 26% of patients had suffered from a persistent sleep-phase delay, which was diagnosed as DSWPD, before the onset of N24SWD. Delayed sleep phase, even in the absence of DSWPD, is highly prevalent in adolescents and young adults,[38] which is consistent with age of onset of N24SWD. As discussed in more detail elsewhere in this article, the interaction between environmental light exposure and internal circadian time may contribute to a common pathway underlying both disorders.

Circadian Rhythm Features

Repeated assessments of strongly endogenous circadian rhythms (eg, melatonin, cortisol, core body temperature) to assess the internal circadian phase or period are rarely performed clinically, but may offer a great deal of insight into the etiology of the disorder and the optimal timing of potential treatment options. When measured, these rhythms tend to exhibit an observed non–24-hour period approximately parallel, although not identical, to the sleep–wake period. The phase angle between the circadian system and the sleep–wake cycle (ie, the timing of sleep relative to internal circadian phase), may be altered in these patients. For example, our previous studies revealed that sleep timing was delayed relative to the melatonin or core body temperature rhythm in patients with N24SWD compared with healthy controls.[39,40] Phase angle disorders likely contribute to the inappropriate light exposure that may underlie the development of N24SWD in some patients and impacts other behaviors, such as mood and performance.

Psychiatric Features

There have been several reports of sighted patients with N24SWD preceded by schizophrenia, bipolar disorder, depression, obsessive–compulsive disorder, or schizoid personality (see **Table 1**). Of the total cohort in the series of sighted patients studied by Hayakawa and colleagues,[6] 28% had developed psychiatric problems before the onset of N24SWD. Kokkoris and colleagues[10] reported on a patient in whom onset of N24SWD was preceded by development of a schizoidlike personality and postulated that this patient's nonentrained sleep–wake pattern was the result of either a primary defect in the mechanism underlying entrainment or weakened social zeitgebers owing to behavioral problems of the personality disorder. Tagaya and colleagues[23] and Wulff and colleagues[41] have also described schizophrenia patients with N24SWD. Although it is possible

that a major defect that prevents circadian entrainment may underlie the sleep disorder, it is more likely for the majority of cases that exposure to inappropriate light–dark cycles induces the nonentrained sleep cycle. The psychiatric disorders and associated medications may induce social withdrawal, behavioral problems, or altered sleep behavior that in turn decrease patients' daytime activities and deprive them of appropriate exposure to sunlight, and/or expose them to unusual artificial light–dark patterns. As discussed elsewhere in this article, self-selected exposure to light can induce a non–24-hour sleep–wake pattern even in healthy subjects.

By contrast, it is indicated that N24SWD may predispose patients to develop psychiatric disorders. In the series from Hayakawa and associates,[6] of those who had no psychiatric problems before the onset of N24SWD, 14 patients (34%) developed major depression thereafter. In 5 of these patients, the symptoms of depression were exacerbated when they slept during the daytime and slightly ameliorated when they slept during the night. This observation suggests that desynchronization between the environmental light–dark cycle and the endogenous circadian phase may increase the risk of developing depression in vulnerable patients.[6] Although reports have indicated that depression is a common psychopathology associated with DSWPD,[42–44] no reports have described systematically the relationship between N24SWD and depression. Phase angle disorders, such as those observed in patients with N24SWD,[39,40] have been associated with a number of depressive disorders (eg,[45–47]) and can determine the time course of mood in healthy, non-depressed subjects (eg,[47–49]). The delay of sleep timing relative to the circadian pacemaker may be an etiologic factor of both the N24SWD[39,40] and the depression that can be associated with N24SWD,[45] the correction of which may be important for long-term treatment of both symptoms.[45]

CLINICAL CHARACTERISTICS OF NON–24-HOUR SLEEP–WAKE RHYTHM DISORDER IN BLIND PATIENTS

Given the central role of light in entraining the circadian pacemaker to the 24-hour day, it is not surprising that those lacking light detection for the circadian system experience problems with maintaining entrainment, and sleep and other rhythm disorders have been recognized in the blind for more than 60 years.[7] Recent studies show that approximately one-half of those with no perception of light exhibit nonentrained circadian rhythms of melatonin, cortisol, or temperature.[7,8,50–52] Many of these patients, but not all, also exhibit non–24-hour sleep–wake rhythms.[53] Although the exact prevalence of N24SWD diagnosed without additional information on other rhythmic variables is unknown, N24SWD is likely to afflict up to two-thirds of the totally blind population. Of the remaining totally blind patients who do not exhibit non–24-hour circadian rhythms, most are entrained to the 24-hour social day (not the 24-hour light–dark cycle) via nonphotic time cues, including strict scheduling of activities, exercise, mealtimes, and social interaction.[51,54,55] In a small proportion of cases (~5%), patients may retain circadian photoreception in the absence of visual function.[56–60] N24SWD in visually impaired patients who retain at least minimal light perception is unusual, with a relatively small number of cases in the literature.[7,8]

Clinical Features

The clinical characteristics of blind patients having N24SWD remain to be formally elucidated. Until recently, the majority of reported cases were male,[51,52,61] although this may simply represent subject selection. A recent study of visually impaired and blind females found that 40% of totally blind females had non–24-hour rhythms, slightly lower than that reported in males.[8,51] Sighted females have a slightly shorter endogenous circadian period than males[62] that, if also true in blind females, as postulated,[63] may increase the proportion of totally blind females with a circadian period closer to 24 hours and therefore more likely to be entrained by nonphotic time cues. A shorter average circadian period would also make it harder to distinguish the period from 24 hours and make the disorder more difficult to detect. There is also a report that race may be associated with circadian period in sighted individuals, with blacks having a slightly shorter period than whites and Asians,[64] which would also theoretically make the disorder more difficult to detect in blacks. Race has not been examined in relation to this disorder in the blind.

Onset can occur at any age, from birth onward,[51,65,66] and usually coincides with or follows shortly after loss of light perception or loss or removal of the eyes.[51]

Type of blindness does not seem to be related to the risk of N24SWD; complete loss of visual and circadian photoreceptive function owing to any ocular disorder will abolish light–dark input to the circadian pacemaker and prevent entrainment to the light–dark cycle. A small proportion of totally visually blind subjects can remain entrained to

the 24-hour light–dark cycle if they retain functional nonrod, noncone, 'nonvisual' photoreception.[56–60] Light detection for circadian entrainment is mediated primarily by a novel nonrod, noncone photoreceptor system located in a small number (<1%) of intrinsically photosensitive retinal ganglion cells. These cells are functionally and anatomically distinct from the traditional rod and cones visual photoreceptors in the outer retina (for reviews, see[67,68]). Disruption of rod and cone function while leaving the ganglion cell layer intact can permit continued light detection for entrainment of the circadian system in the absence of any measurable visual responses and do no result in cyclic sleep–wake disorders.[8,56–60] Eye disorders that damage the ganglion cell layer (eg, glaucoma) or the optic nerve, or removal of the eye entirely (eg, retinoblastoma, trauma) will likely prevent circadian entrainment and increase the likelihood of N24SWD.[7,8,51,52]

Sleep Features

The main sleep features can be similar between sighted and blind patients with N24SWD, namely, a cyclic non–24-hour sleep–wake pattern when measured over several weeks or months, usually with episodes of relatively good sleep followed by episodes of poor nighttime sleep and excessive daytime napping and sleepiness, followed by a return to good sleep ad infinitum.[53] The cyclic nature of the sleep disorder results from the patients' attempt to live on a 24-hour social day while their internal circadian system runs on its non–24-hour intrinsic period. The 2 rhythms run in and out of synchrony with each other such that when the internal circadian rhythm of sleepiness coincides with the social night, sleep is relatively good; when the internal circadian rhythm of sleepiness occurs in the social day, poor nighttime sleep and high levels of daytime sleepiness phase ensue. If the patient lived on a non–24-hour "day length" equal to their internal circadian period, a sleep disorder would not be apparent (eg, **Fig. 2**C, b).

As illustrated in **Fig. 2**, nighttime sleep is most often attempted at a normal social time, and sleep onset and offset times occur across a relatively narrow range (≤3 hours). Nighttime sleep and daytime nap duration tend to vary reciprocally according the circadian phase at which nighttime sleep is attempted. When nighttime sleep coincides with the peak production of melatonin at night, nighttime duration is maximal and daytime naps minimal. This situation is reversed when nighttime sleep is attempted when melatonin production occurs during the

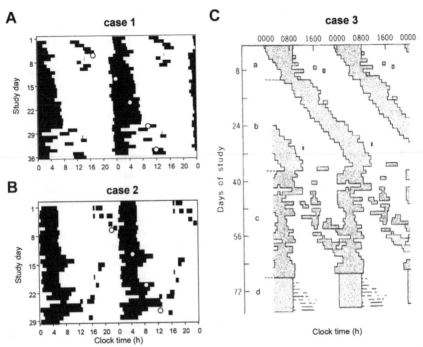

Fig. 2. Non–24-hour sleep–wake rhythm disorder in 3 totally blind men plotted as in **Fig. 1**. The peak time of the urinary 6-sulphatoxymelatonin rhythm, collected each week, is also plotted (○ in A and B). (A) Case 1 is a 66-year-old totally blind man with 1 eye and no conscious light perception owing to ocular trauma. He exhibits a non–24-hour sleep–wake cycle and a melatonin rhythm with a period (τ) of 24.68 hours. (B) Case 2 is a 35-year-old bilaterally enucleated (retinoblastoma) man who also has a 24.68-hour melatonin rhythm and N24SWD. Both patients exhibit the characteristic recurrent episodes of disturbed nighttime sleep and many daytime naps when nighttime sleep is attempted at an adverse circadian phase (ie, when melatonin peaks during the day; eg, case 1, days 1–8 or 28–35) that alternates with episodes of good sleep at night when it coincides with nighttime melatonin production (eg, case 1, days 10–25). (C) Case 3 shows the sleep–wake pattern of a 28-year-old man who lost his light perception at birth owing to retinopathy of prematurity (retrolental fibroplasia). Sections a and c represent his sleep while living freely at home and section b shows sleep during an ad lib inpatient study when the subject was free to sleep as he pleased. During section d, an unsuccessful attempt was made to entrain his cycle via strict 24-hour scheduling of sleep, meals and activity. While living freely in the laboratory (b), his sleep–wake, plasma cortisol, alertness, performance, and urinary electrolyte rhythms all exhibited a circadian period of 24.9 hours. This rhythm persisted when living at home (c) but was modulated by attempting to live on a social 24-hour day, as in cases 1 and 2 (ie, exhibited relative coordination; see text). (Cases 1 and 2 *reproduced from* Lockley SW. Sleep, melatonin and other circadian rhythms in the blind. PhD thesis, University of Surrey, Guildford, UK. Case 3 *from* Miles LE, Raynal DM, Wilson MA. Blind man living in normal society has circadian rhythms of 24.9 hours. Science 1977;198(4315):422; with permission.

day. The melatonin rhythm can be considered marker of the biological night, or the time at which the circadian drive for sleepiness is maximal. When sleep occurs outside this time, sleep duration, timing, and quality are impaired[53] and patients experience daytime dysfunction in their sleepiness, mood, and performance.[69] There is a lot of variability in the expression of sleep phenotypes in blind patients with nonentrained circadian rhythms, however, with the majority of patients exhibiting subtle changes in their sleep which require prolonged assessment to detect.[70]

The longitudinal polysomnographic measurements required to observe the cyclic nature of

the disruptions to sleep structure have also not typically been performed in totally blind patients. One case study[71] has quantified detailed changes in sleep structure and showed changes consistent with laboratory studies of sleep in healthy, sighted subjects at different circadian phases.[36,72] Single-night recordings of nonentrained totally blind subjects also show changes in sleep structure consistent with some of them sleeping at an adverse circadian phase,[61,73] although without additional longitudinal assessments, single-night polysomnographic measures are difficult to interpret.

When assessed over many weeks or months, the cyclic nature of the sleep disturbance is easier to detect.[53,74,75] **Fig. 2**A, B shows representative examples of self-reported sleep–wake records in 2 totally blind patients with N24SWD; a 66-year-old man and a 35-year-old man. Cases 1 and 2 had a nonentrained rhythm of 24.68 hours in urinary 6-sulphatoxymelatonin, the major urinary metabolite of melatonin (see **Fig. 2**A, B, ○; S20 and S31, respectively[51]). Their average night-sleep duration (6.2 and 5.8 hours, respectively) and total sleep time per 24 hours (7.2 and 6.3 hours, respectively) are typical of blind patients with N24SWD, which is usually reduced compared with blind subjects with normally phase circadian rhythms.[53] Case 3 represents the first detailed case report of N24SWD in a blind subject[74] and shows a 28-year-old man with a 24.9-hour rhythm in sleep, plasma cortisol, and other parameters. When living freely, the 24.9-hour sleep rhythm is clearly observed (see **Fig. 2**C, b), but changes, as seen cases 1 and 2, when attempting to live on a social 24-hour day (see **Fig. 2**C, c), with the characteristic changes in nighttime and daytime sleep described[53]; clear "relative coordination" of the sleep–wake pattern occurs as the 24-hour social schedule cycles in and out of phase with the internal non–24-hour circadian system.

Circadian Rhythm Features

As illustrated, non–24-hour circadian rhythm disorders in the blind have tended to be confirmed from circadian markers other than sleep, such as melatonin or cortisol rhythms.[7,8,50–52,76] Collectively, these studies show that circadian rhythms in totally blind subjects can be categorized into 4 main groups: normal circadian phase, advanced phase, delayed phase, and non–24-hour nonentrained rhythms. Of these, nonentrained subjects are the largest group, representing 40% to 60% of totally blind patients with individual circadian periods ranging from 23.8 to 25.1 hours. The remainder are divided approximately equally between normal and abnormally phased (advanced or delayed) rhythms. It is possible that some of these subjects are misclassified and actually represent nonentrained rhythms with a period very close to, and difficult to distinguish from, 24 hours.[56] As discussed, some totally visually blind patients do remain entrained to 24 hours either via nonphotic time cues or intact circadian photoreception.

Given the social restraints on the sleep–wake pattern, the non–24-hour sleep–wake rhythm is often not as readily observed as other nonsleep rhythms.[53,70] The observed period of the sleep–wake cycle is usually shorter than that of the hormonal rhythms, if apparent at all. For example, of 16 totally blind subjects with nonentrained melatonin rhythms (range, 24.1–24.8 hours), only 7 had non–24-hour activity rhythms and only 5 had non–24-hour sleep rhythms (<24.3 hours; see Fig. 1 in ref[53]). Similarly, one-quarter of these patients did not complain of sleep disturbance (as assessed using the Pittsburgh Sleep Quality Index[51]).

This apparent inconsistency may occur for several reasons. Most people do not sleep precisely according to their circadian phase given strong social cues to do otherwise (eg, school, work, family commitments) and often use stimulants to overcome this nonoptimal sleep as illustrated by the very wide use of caffeine. Blind patients with a short circadian period only change their internal circadian phase by a few minutes per day and may not recognize minor changes to sleep as part of a cyclic sleep disorder. For example, a patient with a circadian period of 24.1 hours has a 6-minute internal change per day that may be relatively easy to overcome in the short term. Because it takes a very long number of days to complete a full circadian cycle and free-run "around the clock" (121 days, or 4 months, if the period = 24.1 hours), neither patient nor physician would recognize the sleep disorder as cyclic and may diagnose insomnia owing to the poor sleep when maximally out of phase. A patient with a period of 24.67 hours, however, would have a shift of 40 minutes per day in internal time and a much more noticeable change in their ability to sleep (35 days to complete 1 circadian cycle). These patients often readily recognize that their sleep changes from day to day in a predictable manner and are easier to diagnose as having N24SWD. Most patients do not have such a clear phenotype and exhibit a subtle relative coordination or episodic sleep complaint that is not apparent without prolonged records.[70] Even without a sleep complaint, patients with non–24-hour circadian rhythms may still exhibit cyclic sleep–wake patterns and may benefit from treatment to improve both their sleep and daytime functioning. These data illustrate the vital importance of assessing strong circadian markers in addition to sleep to diagnose correctly N24SWD. It is not known if there are sighted individuals who also have a similar phenotype, namely a non–24-hour internal pacemaker but with a near-normal sleep–wake cycle. Such people would not seek treatment and would presumably be relatively rare.

Psychiatric Features

The detailed reports of circadian rhythm sleep disorders in blind patients have excluded those with psychiatric disorders before study; therefore, little is known about the psychiatric features of blind patients with N24SWD. Noncyclic sleep disorders are common in visually impaired patients,[77–79] which have been suggested to be owing, at least in part, to concomitant psychiatric disorders.[79]

BIOLOGICAL BASIS AND PATHOGENESIS OF NON–24-HOUR SLEEP–WAKE RHYTHM DISORDER

Non–24-hour sleep–wake rhythm disorder occurs because the internal circadian pacemaker and sleep–wake cycle do not remain entrained with the 24-hour light–dark cycle. In totally blind patients, the reason for lack of entrainment to the light–dark cycle is clear. In sighted subjects with N24SWD, the exact mechanisms responsible for this desynchrony are unknown, but are likely to be multiple in origin (**Fig. 3**). In particular, an abnormal interaction between the endogenous circadian rhythm and the sleep homeostatic process that regulates sleep and wakefulness plays an essential role in the pathophysiology of N24SWD.[5,80] The biological factors possibly related to the pathogenesis of N24SWD are reviewed briefly.

Phase Angle Difference Between the Circadian Pacemaker and Sleep–Wake Cycle

Under normal conditions, most people tend to go to sleep at a particular circadian phase that corresponds with the rising part of the melatonin rhythm and the falling limb of the core body temperature cycle. If the core body temperature minimum, or

trough, is used as a nominal circadian phase marker, most people tend to initiate sleep onset approximately 4 to 6 hours before, and wake 2 to 3 hours after body temperature minimum (**Fig. 4**). Under conditions of temporal isolation, but with self-timed access to light, subjects tend initiate sleep at a later circadian phase, closer to their body temperature minimum.[4,64] The body temperature minimum happens to coincide with a particularly sensitive part of the circadian cycle, namely the phase at which light changes from causing a phase delay of the circadian pacemaker (shifting to a later time) to causing a phase advance (shifting to an earlier time). The magnitude and direction of the phase resetting effects of light is described more fully by several phase response curves (PRC).[81–84] By initiating sleep at a later circadian phase, individuals "expose" more of their PRC to the delaying effects of light and reduce exposure at a time when advances would occur when they close their eyes to sleep or switch off the light, resulting in a net daily phase delay.[5,39,85] Under these conditions, subjects exhibit a long circadian "period," often 25 hours or more, as a result of the daily net delays owing to the self-selected exposure to light. The resulting sleep–wake pattern is very similar to that exhibited by sighted patients with N24SWD, including a long non–24-hour circadian period and recurrent phase delay jumps and long sleep episodes when the sleep timing is initiated at a particular circadian phase (**Fig. 5**, middle panel[85]). When subjects are studied in an environment free of time cues but with light–dark

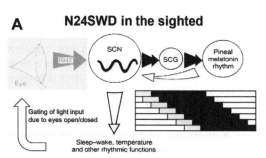
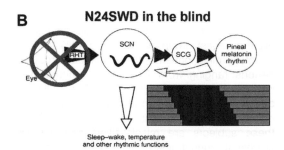

Fig. 3. Anatomic basis of sleep and circadian rhythm disruption. Mechanisms that compromise circadian organization may underlie non–24-hour sleep–wake rhythm disorder (N24SWD) in the sighted (*A*) and blind (*B*). The basic organization of the circadian system comprises 3 parts; an endogenous near–24-hour oscillator located in the suprachiasmatic nuclei (SCN) that is synchronized via light–dark input from the retinaretinohypothalamic tract (RHT) –SCN pathway, which then sends efferent signals to the pineal gland and other brain areas to control the timing of melatonin and sleep–wake rhythms, respectively, among others. (*A*) In sighted patients with N24SWD, the endogenous circadian pacemaker is intact and functional, but is likely systematically phase delayed by inappropriate exposure to light, resulting in a sleep–wake cycle of approximately 25 hours. (*B*) In blind patients, the pacemaker is also functionally intact but reverts to its near 24-hour endogenous periodicity (~24.5 hours) owing to a nonfunctional RHT. N24SWD, non–24-hour sleep–wake rhythm disorder. (*Adapted from* Lockley SW, Cohen D, Harper DG, et al. Other circadian rhythm disorders: Non-24-hour sleep-wake disorder and irregular sleep-wake disorder. [Book Chapter]. In: Barkoukis T, Matheson JK, Ferber R, et al, editors. Therapy in sleep medicine. Amsterdam (The Netherlands): Elsevier; 2011. p. 417; with permission.)

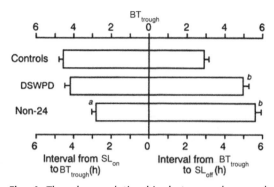

Fig. 4. The phase relationship between sleep and circadian phase in circadian rhythm sleep disorders. The graph shows the intervals from sleep onset to body temperature (BT) trough (BT_{trough}) and from BT_{trough} to sleep offset in control subjects, delayed sleep wake phase disorder (DSWPD) patients, and non–24-hour sleep–wake syndrome (N24SWD) patients. The time interval from sleep onset (SL_{on}) to BT_{trough} is significantly shorter and the time from BT_{trough} to sleep offset (SL_{off}) is significantly longer in the N24SWD patients than in the controls and DSWPD patients, meaning that N24SWD patients go to sleep and wake later in their circadian cycle. This abnormal phase relationship between the sleep and circadian rhythms exposes N24SWD patients to more light at a time that will cause a phase delay of their circadian pacemaker and decreases light exposure at a time that would cause a corrective phase advance. DSWPD, delayed sleep-wake rhythm disorder; Non-24, non–24-hour sleep–wake rhythm disorder. (*From* Uchiyama M, Okawa M, Shibui K, et al. Altered phase relation between sleep timing and core body temperature rhythm in delayed sleep phase syndrome and non–24-hour sleep–wake syndrome in humans. Neurosci Lett 2000;294:103; with permission.)

exposure scheduled to a 20- or 28-hour day, the circadian period observed is much closer to 24 hours (on average 24.2 hours; see **Fig. 5**) and likely represents more accurately the intrinsic period of the circadian pacemaker.[85]

Detailed studies of the timing of sleep relative to the body temperature minimum or melatonin rhythm in patients with DSWPS and N24SWD[5,6,39,40,86] show that these patients also tend to initiate sleep at a later circadian phase compared with normal controls, with N24SWD patients initiating sleep later than DSWPS patients (see **Fig. 4**).[39] The timing of the sleep behavior may indicate a common basis between what happens to humans under temporal isolation and the pathophysiology of these circadian rhythm disorders. By sleeping at a relatively late circadian phase, and for a relatively long duration,[39] patients expose themselves to light and avoid light at times that causes a net phase delay each day, inducing a non–24-hour sleep–wake cycle. The

underlying cause of this late sleep time may be owing to an inherent internal desynchronization between the sleep–wake homeostat and the circadian system,[80,85] and preliminary studies suggest that patients with N24SWD may have difficulty in increasing homeostatic sleep pressure.[40,87] A more likely cause of the disorder is a change in behavior whereby patients choose to sleep later in their circadian cycle and induce a systematic phase delay. This explanation may also account for the observation that DSWPD often precedes N24SWD and that a DSWPD-like sleep pattern and a N24SWD-like sleep pattern can be observed in the same patient.[6] Consistent with this hypothesis, Emens and colleagues[24] reported that a sighted patient suffering from N24SWD with a sleep–wake cycle of 25.17 hours under a normal 24-hour day–night condition displayed a core body temperature rhythm of 24.5 hours under a forced desynchrony protocol, suggesting that self-selected access to light artificially lengthened his observed circadian period. The association between N24SWD and psychiatric disorders further supports the idea that unusual behavior may initiate and then drive the development of N24SWD.

Decreased Circadian Phase Resetting Response to Light

Although the circadian resetting effect of light is abolished in totally blind patients with N24SWD, sighted subjects may theoretically suffer from an impaired response to light resetting that prevents appropriate entrainment with the light–dark cycle. A blunted response to light-induced melatonin suppression test as a proxy marker for sensitivity to circadian light responses has been reported in 2 single-case studies,[26,28] but an attenuated phase shifting response has not been confirmed. Differences in individual PRCs, such as a decreased sensitivity in the phase advancing portion of the PRC, could also hypothetically underlie the disorder, as could impairments in circadian photoreception (eg, melanopsin dysfunction) in the presence of normal vision, although there are no reports of such patients in the literature.

Longer Endogenous Circadian Period

Only 1 study has studied systematically the endogenous circadian period of sighted patients with N24SWD. Kitamura and colleagues,[88] using a forced desynchrony protocol with 28-hour sleep–wake schedule, examined the endogenous circadian period of 6 sighted N24SWD patients and 17 healthy controls (intermediate and evening chronotypes). The τ of the patients (24.48 hours) was significantly longer than that of combined

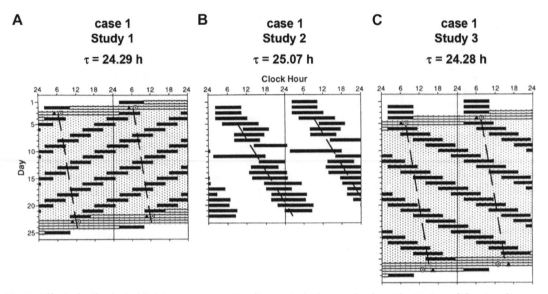

Fig. 5. Effect of self-selected light exposure on circadian period. The graphs show the timing of the circadian system in a single subject studied under 3 different laboratory conditions. In studies 1 and 3 (*A* and *C*, respectively), the subject was scheduled to live on a 20- and 28-hour sleep–wake/light–dark cycle, respectively, with sleep only permitted for one-third of each "day" (■). During scheduled wake times, light was kept relatively dim (<15 lux). These forced desynchrony protocols are outside the limits of entrainment for the circadian pacemaker and the clock reverts to its endogenous period, as illustrated by the fact that the circadian system has the same period (τ = 24.28 hours, *dashed line*) for the body temperature rhythm under both the 20- and 28-hour protocols. When the same subject was allowed to live freely (*B*, study 2) and choose when to sleep and when to switch on normal room lights (*middle panel*; 150 lux), the temperature rhythm had a longer period (τ = 25.07 hours; *dashed line*) and the sleep pattern resembled that of patients with non–24-hour sleep–wake syndrome (see **Fig. 1**). The sleep–wake cycle "free-ran" with a long period (27.07 hours) and had characteristic "phase jumps" as the sleep onset time approached the morning hours. The gradual change in when sleep occurs relative to the body temperature minimum (*dashed line*) is clear, with sleep onset occurring closer and closer to the body temperature minimum. Light exposure before the body temperature minimum causes a phase delay of the circadian pacemaker (see text) and is progressively delaying the circadian pacemaker, inducing the non–24-hour sleep–wake rhythm disorder. (*From* Czeisler CA, Duffy JF, Shanahan TL, et al. Stability, precision, and near-24-hour period of the human circadian pacemaker. Science 1999;284(5423):2177–81; with permission.)

healthy controls (24.17 hours) and that of the intermediate chronotypes (24.12 hours), but was not statistically different from that of evening chronotypes potentially given the high variance in circadian period of evening chronotypes. Moreover, the circadian period of the melatonin rhythm in N24SWD patients was not correlated with that of the sleep–wake cycles observed before the study, consistent with an earlier case study,[24] and concluded that although a longer τ may be implicated in the onset mechanism of N24SWD, it is not the only factor involved. In animal studies, mutations of core clock genes that cause expression of an abnormally long or short endogenous circadian period have been shown to be responsible for alteration of the phase angle between the rest–activity cycle and the 24-hour environmental light–dark cycle.[89,90] A number of reports have associated mutations and polymorphisms in circadian clock genes with advanced sleep–wake phase disorder and DSWPD (reviewed in[91]),

including a relatively short circadian period in a woman with severe advanced sleep–wake rhythm disorder.[92] More recently, 2 studies have examined potential genetic polymorphisms that underlie N24SWD. Hida and colleagues[93] genotyped single nucleotide polymorphisms in circadian clock genes in N24SWD individuals, DSWPD individuals, and controls, and found that the PER3 polymorphism (rs228697) was significantly associated with diurnal preference and the N24SWD phenotype, and that the minor allele of rs228697 was more prevalent in evening types than in morning types and in N24SWD individuals compared with the controls, suggesting that PER3 polymorphisms could be a potential genetic marker for an individual's circadian and sleep phenotypes. Kripke and colleagues[94] undertook a substudy of sighted N24SWD patients within a larger assessment of circadian clock genes in DSWPD. Of 38 patients with suspected non–24-hour sleep–wake rhythms based on actigraphy, 3 were considered to have definite non–24-hour sleep cycles and all 3 were heterozygous for the C (minor) allele of rs908078, as was another participant with a possible non–24-hour component and 6 with DSWPD. They concluded that several circadian gene loci promoted phase delay, probably including the associated allele pattern of BHLHE40, which was also associated with non–24-hour sleep–wake cycles.[94]

TREATMENT STRATEGIES FOR NON–24-HOUR SLEEP–WAKE RHYTHM DISORDER

Therapeutic interventions for N24SWD should be targeted at entraining the patient's circadian pacemaker at an appropriate phase relative to the environmental light–dark cycle. Although light exposure or administration of melatonin and its analogs have been shown to reset the phase of the circadian pacemaker in sighted healthy subjects

and some patient groups, there have been no large-scale, controlled trials for treating N24SWD in sighted patients; therefore, treatment options are based largely on case studies at this time. In the totally blind, melatonin has been shown to reset the circadian clock and, recently, 2 phase III clinical trials of tasimelteon (Vanda Pharmaceuticals, Inc), a dual melatonin receptor agonist, to treat N24SWD in the totally blind were recently completed and have led to approval of tasimelteon to treat N24SWD in the blind in the United States and Europe. These strategies are reviewed elsewhere in this article.

Light Therapy

In humans and other mammals, appropriately timed exposure to light can reset the phase of circadian rhythms.[81–84] As has been reviewed, the most sensitive phase of PRC to light usually coincides with the last one-half of the sleep

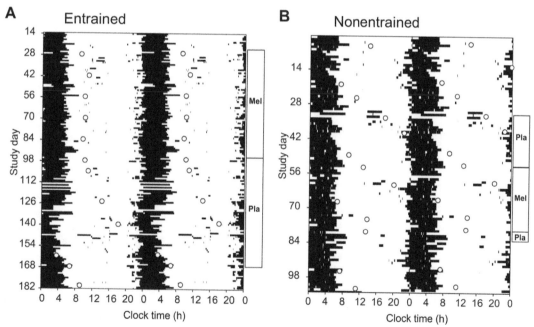

Fig. 6. Melatonin treatment of non–24-hour sleep–wake rhythm disorder in the blind. The graphs show double-plotted sleep timing (■) and urinary cortisol peak times (○) for 2 totally blind men treated with 5 mg fast-release melatonin (MEL) orally at 21:00 hours over at least 1 circadian cycle. Sequential study days are plotted on the ordinate and clock time is quadruple-plotted on the abscissa. The study had a placebo-controlled, single-blind design[97] and the start and end of placebo (PLA) and MEL treatment are indicated by the adjacent boxes. (A) A subject who was entrained by MEL treatment (S17). He exhibited a nonentrained cortisol rhythm (24.3 hours) during PLA treatment but was entrained at a normal circadian phase by the MEL treatment (mean ± SD cortisol peak time = 9.9 ± 0.7 hours). The entrained sleep–wake cycle observed during MEL treatment becomes immediately disrupted upon cessation of treatment and reverts to the characteristic non–24-hour cyclic pattern. (B) A subject who failed to entrain to 5 mg MEL treatment (S45) despite receiving treatment for nearly 2 full circadian cycles. The persistent cyclic non–24-hour sleep–wake rhythm disorder is clearly apparent throughout both the PLA and MEL treatment. (*From* Lockley SW, Arendt J, Skene DJ. Visual impairment and circadian rhythm disorders. Dialogues Clin Neurosci 2007;9(3):310.)

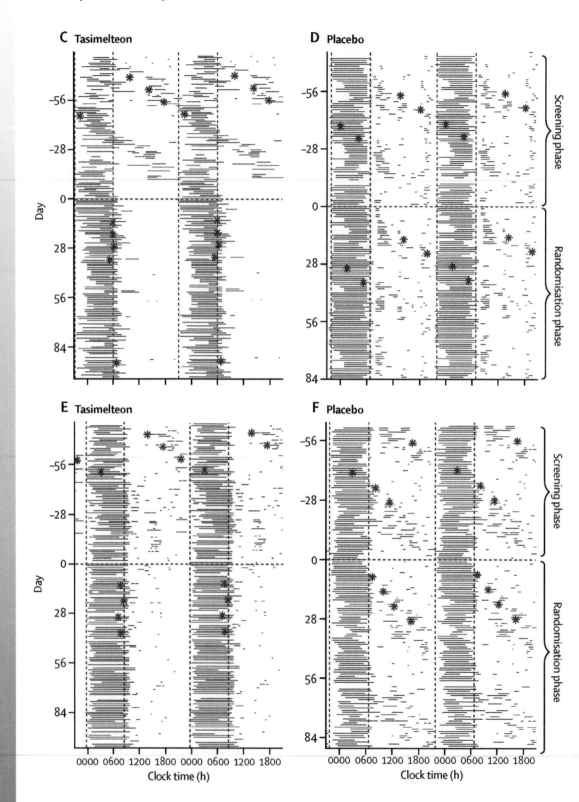

episode, and therefore the timing of the sleep itself is a major determinant of light input to the pacemaker. If self-selected light exposure is the underlying cause of the disorders, behavioral therapy aimed at correcting unusual sleep–wake behavior may be useful. Direct light therapy for N24SWD has been used in a number of cases with the aim of inducing a phase advance of the circadian pacemaker to counteract the typical phase delay observed (eg,[13,17,31,33]). The initial timing of light therapy relative to the patients' internal circadian pacemaker may be key in ensuring that the light therapy does not exacerbate the adverse circadian phase by causing a phase shift opposite to that required. Lighting exposure timed to advance the clock should start after the body temperature minimum, and light should be avoided before body temperature minimum to decrease phase-delaying effects. Clinical measurement of circadian phase for diagnosis or treatment timing is rarely performed, but can be achieved relatively simply using home-based assessments of salivary or urinary melatonin timing and its metabolites.[51,95,96] In the absence of circadian phase information, asking the patient to maintain a fixed rise time and performing morning light therapy at the same time for several weeks, so that eventually the light therapy is applied during the phase-advance portion of the PRC, may be successful.

Melatonin Treatment

Appropriately timed melatonin can also phase shift the human circadian pacemaker, with the pattern of the melatonin PRC broadly opposite to that of light; under normally entrained conditions, melatonin administered in the early evening induces a phase advance, and in the early morning, a phase delay.[98] Melatonin also has sleepiness-inducing properties in addition to its ability to shift the circadian pacemaker[99] and, therefore, the time of administration should also take this into account. Sighted patients with N24SWD have been treated successfully in open-label studies of melatonin therapy,[26,31,100] although no controlled clinical trials have been published. As with light therapy, prior knowledge of circadian phase is important for timing treatment appropriately. To phase advance the internal pacemaker optimally, melatonin treatment needs to be administered at or before the onset of the rise in melatonin production (termed the dim light melatonin onset[95,96]). Without prior knowledge of circadian phase, maintaining melatonin treatment at a fixed time in the early evening for several weeks may provide some benefit.

Use of melatonin treatment for N24SWD in blind patients has been more studied extensively, although still in a relatively small number of

Fig. 7. Tasimelteon treatment of non–24-hour sleep–wake rhythm disorder in the blind. **Fig. 7** illustrates the pattern of subjective nighttime and daytime sleep (start to end of each sleep episode; black *lines*) and acrophases derived from serial 48-hour measures of urinary 6-sulfatoxymelatonin (aMT6s; red stars) for 4 totally blind patients enrolled in SET. Sequential study days during screening (S-, *shaded area*) and from randomization (day 0) are shown on the ordinate axis and clock time is double-plotted on the abscissa. Self-selected 9-hour sleep opportunities are denoted by the vertical gray dotted lines and treatment was scheduled 1 hour before scheduled bedtime at a fixed clock time. Two patients exhibited clear non–24-hour rhythms before treatment (patient D, 68 years old, $\tau = 24.71 \pm 0.16$ hours; patient F, 64 years old, $\tau = 24.67 \pm 0.19$ hours), and placebo treatment did not change their circadian period (post-treatment $\tau = 24.73 \pm 0.23$ hours and 24.41 ± 0.15 hours, respectively). There was also no significant change in the lowest quartile of nighttime total sleep time (LQ-nTST change from screening to treatment of 3.54 to 4.25 hours, and from 3.04 to 3.08 hours, respectively), or upper quartile of the duration of total daytime sleep (UQ-dTSD change from 2.82 to 2.70 hours, and from 3.50 to 3.27 hours, respectively) and were rated unchanged in a Clinical Global Impression of Change assessment (CGI-C = 5.0 and 3.5, respectively; 7-point scale, from 1 [very much improved] to 7 [very much worse]). (*C, E*) Two patients who entrained to 20 mg tasimelteon treatment. Patient C (44 years old) was not entrained ($\tau = 24.59 \pm 0.07$ hours) and had substantial sleep disruption (LQ-nTST = 1.35 hours, UQ-dTSD = 3.69 hours) during screening but following tasimelteon treatment, became stably entrained ($\tau = 24.01 \pm 0.01$ hours; mean aMT6s acrophase = 6:07 AM) and had improved nighttime and daytime sleep during the worst quartile by 142 and 182 min/d, respectively (LQ-nTST = 3.72 hours, UQ-dTSD = 0.66 hours; CGI-C = 1.5). Patient E (31 years old) was also entrained by tasimelteon (τ changed from 24.58 ± 0.10 hours to 24.00 ± 0.08 hours; aMT6s acrophase = 7:34 AM), and exhibited improvements in nighttime (LQ-nTST) and daytime (UQ-dTSD) sleep by 101 and 79 min/d, and had a CGI-C rating of 2.0. The interindividual variability in the severity and cyclicity of the nighttime and daytime sleep disruption is apparent, although when assessed over several months, reliable cyclic disorders appear. The pattern of aMT6s timing is sufficient to detect non–24-hour rhythms in several weeks, however. (*From* Lockley SW, Dressman MA, Licamele L, et al. Tasimelteon for non–24-hour sleep–wake disorder in totally blind people (SET and RESET): two multicentre, randomised, double-masked, placebo-controlled phase 3 trials. Lancet, in press; with permission.)

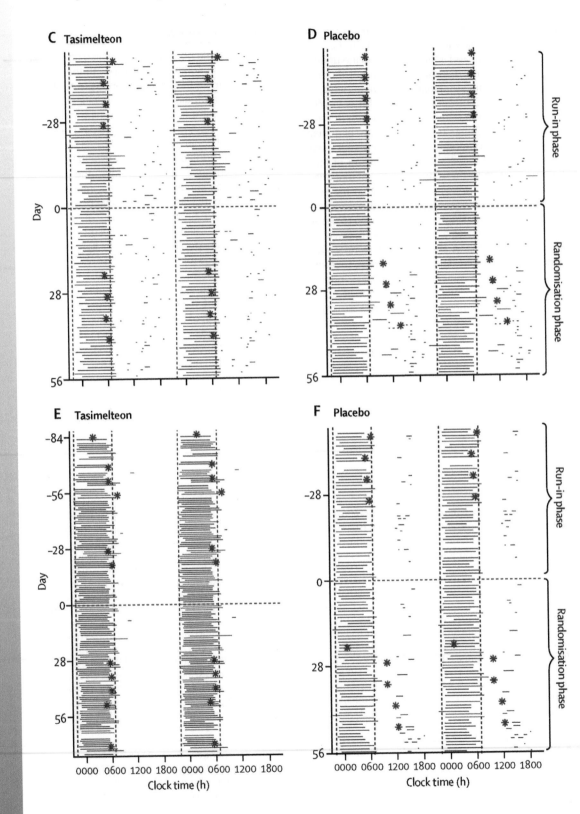

patients.[7] Although the soporific properties of melatonin have been shown to "stabilize" the sleep–wake cycle in blind patients without entrainment of the circadian pacemaker,[101] entrainment of the circadian pacemaker, and therefore the sleep rhythm, is necessary to treat N24SWD fully. After the initial demonstrations that a 5-mg[97] or 10-mg[73] dose could entrain circadian rhythms in the blind, several studies have shown that lower doses ($\leq$0.5 mg) seem to be equally as effective, if not more so,[102,103] at entraining the clock maybe through providing a more discreet temporal signal than higher doses. Given melatonin's soporific properties, treatment should be administered at the same time each day, close to the desired bedtime to ensure the alignment of the circadian and social day. Although a 2-mg, prolonged-release preparation of melatonin was reported to improve sleep in blind patients with sleep complaints (but without a confirmed nonentrained clock),[104] its prolonged release profile makes this preparation an unlikely candidate to provide the discreet 24-hour time cue required to reset the circadian clock each day owing to potential (ie, persistent blood concentrations would likely mean that the drug would be present and "spillover" both the advance and delay portions of the PRC).[98,105]

Regarding the circadian time of administration, although low doses ($\leq$0.5 mg) initiated at any circadian phase eventually cause entrainment of the circadian pacemaker,[102,103,105–107] there may be a lag in experiencing beneficial effects until the time of administration coincides with the phase advance part of the PRC. If treatment can be timed initially to induce a phase advance, entrainment should occur within a few days and the patient will perceive immediate benefit (**Fig. 6**). The

individuals' circadian period may also affect the likelihood of entrainment with melatonin,[108] because those subjects with periods furthest from 24 hours may be outside the range of entrainment for this relatively weak time cue. Long-term safety data are not available for melatonin, although research studies suggest that it is a relatively safe drug in most patient groups.[109,110]

Melatonin Agonist Treatment

Recently, 2 placebo-controlled, randomized, double-masked phase III trials of 20 mg tasimelteon, a melatonin MT1/MT2 agonist,[111,112] were conducted in totally blind adult patients (18–75 years) with sleep complaints and confirmed non–24-hour rhythms in urinary aMT6s ($\tau \geq$24.25 hours).[113]

The Safety and Efficacy of Tasimelteon (SET) study (n = 84) showed that daily tasimelteon treatment (fixed clock time 1 hour before fixed target bedtime) for 6 months could entrain the circadian clock and improve clinical measures of nighttime and daytime sleep compared with placebo (**Fig. 7**). The Randomized withdrawal on the Efficacy and Safety of Tasimelteon (RESET) study (n = 20) showed that, once patients were entrained with tasimelteon, treatment had to be continued to maintain circadian entrainment and the associated clinical benefits, because withdrawal to placebo permitted the clock to return to its non–24-hour rhythm (**Fig. 8**). Tasimelteon was safe and well-tolerated.[113] These clinical studies form the basis of the data that led to approval of tasimelteon to treat N24SWD by the US Food and Drug Administration and the European Medicines Agency.

◄────────────────────────

Fig. 8. Tasimelteon withdrawal after treatment of non–24-hour our sleep–wake rhythm disorder in the blind. The graph shows patients who were enrolled in RESET (see **Fig. 7** for legend). Treatment was scheduled at a fixed clock time 1 hour before scheduled bedtime throughout. All patients received tasimelteon before randomization in an open-label run-in and all 4 patients show clear entrainment of the 6-sulfatoxymelatonin (aMT6s) acrophase (mean range, 6:14 AM–7:25 AM) during run-in and stable, noncyclic nighttime sleep with few daytime naps. At randomization (day 0), patients were randomized to continued tasimelteon treatment or withdrawn to placebo in a double-masked manner. When patients were withdrawn from treatment (patients D and F), the pacemaker reverted to its non–24-hour period (τ = 24.19 $\pm$ 0.17 hours and 24.13 $\pm$ 0.09 hours, respectively) and the clinical consequences reemerged. In patient D, nighttime sleep (lowest quartile of nighttime total sleep time [LQ-nTST]) worsened by an average of 199 minutes per night and daytime sleep (upper quartile of the duration of total daytime sleep [UQ-dTSD]) increased by 44 minutes per day compared with run-in, and the disruptive cyclic sleep patterns returned. Patient F had similarly worsened sleep, with 32 minutes less sleep per night (LQ-nTST) and 33 minutes more sleep per day (UQ-dTSD) after cessation of treatment. When tasimelteon treatment is maintained (patients C and E), entrainment is maintained (τ = 24.03 $\pm$ 0.07 hours and 23.99 $\pm$ 0.03 hours, respectively; aMT6s acrophase mean, patient G = 5:37 AM, patient H = 5:34 AM) along with the clinical benefits (patient C; LQ-nTST increase of 19 minutes per day; UQ-dTSD decrease of 21 minutes per day; patient E; LQ-nTST decrease of 43 minutes per day; UQ-dTSD change of 1 minute per day). (From Lockley SW, Dressman MA, Licamele L, et al. Tasimelteon for non–24-hour sleep–wake disorder in totally blind people (SET and RESET): two multicentre, randomised, double-masked, placebo-controlled phase 3 trials. Lancet, in press; with permission.)

Other Compounds

Combined therapies have been tried in case studies of sighted patients with reported success, including use of the melatonin agonist, ramelteon (Takeda Pharmaceuticals) combined with methyl-cobalamin (a vitamin B_{12} preparation), light manipulation, and triazolam[114]; vitamin B_{12} with light therapy and or hypnotics[14,115]; and modafinil in combination with light and melatonin therapy.[116] Although sleep seems to be stabilized in these cases, it is not clear if the circadian clock is reset, and the underlying clock disorder treated, as non-sleep outcomes are typically not measured.

Several case studies have also examined whether other compounds can entrain the non–24-hour clock in blind patients including triazolam[117] or caffeine,[118] without success. Morning caffeine administration does improve daytime alertness ratings, particularly at an adverse circadian phase, but does not address the underlying circadian disorder.[118]

SUMMARY

More detailed assessments of sleep and circadian rhythms in N24SWD, under both field and laboratory conditions, will improve the diagnosis and treatment of this disorder. Given the variability in the presentation of sleep phenotypes in N24SWD, we need to use more reliable measures of the circadian clock such as melatonin and cortisol in clinical practice, and formal guidelines are needed to inform physicians how to measure and interpret these data.[1,2]

The approval of tasimelteon to treat N24SWD in the totally blind is a major breakthrough in the field, not only for patients, but also because it is the first treatment approved for any disorder that relies on resetting of the circadian clock, as opposed to simply treating the symptoms of a circadian rhythm disorder, such as insomnia or excessive sleepiness. The use of circadian entrainment as a clinical trial endpoint is also an important step forward, because it introduces the concept of shifting or resetting the clock as important in its own right within the medical establishment, in addition to symptomatic relief. A similar approach is needed for sighted patients with N24SWD, and large-scale clinical trials are required to establish the risk factors and treatment guidelines.

DISCLOSURE STATEMENT

Dr M. Uchiyama has received research support from Astellas Pharma, Eisai, Meiji Seika Pharma, MSD, Pfizer Japan, Taisho Pharmaceutical, Kao Corporation, and Takeda Pharmaceutical, and has consulted for Pfizer Japan, Kao Corporation, Taisho Pharmaceutical and Takeda Pharmaceutical. He has also received honoraria for giving lectures and/or contributing text from Astellas Pharma, Eisai, Otsuka Pharmaceutical, Meiji Seika Pharma, MSD, and Takeda Pharmaceutical. Dr S.W. Lockley was the principal investigator of 3 recently completed clinical trials of a melatonin agonist for the treatment of non–24-hour sleep–wake disorder in the blind, sponsored by Vanda Pharmaceuticals. Inc, and has received an investigator-initiated research grant and 2 service agreements from Vanda Pharmaceuticals, Inc, related to non–24-hour rhythms in the blind. He has also received minor consulting fees from 15 financial companies related to non–24-hour sleep–wake disorder in the blind and the publicly available clinical trial results. He has also received honoraria from MediCom Worldwide, Inc, for teaching on a CME course sponsored by Vanda Pharmaceuticals, Inc; for contributing text about non–24-hour sleep–wake disorder for the National Sleep Foundation and textbook chapters published by Elsevier; and in 2007 received an authorship fees from Servier Inc, for writing a review of circadian rhythm disorders in the blind.

REFERENCES

1. American Academy of Sleep Medicine. International classification of sleep disorders: diagnostic and coding manual. 3rd edition. Darien (IL): America Academy of Sleep Medicine; 2014.
2. Sack RL, Auckley D, Auger RR, et al. Circadian rhythm sleep disorders: part II, advanced sleep phase disorder, delayed sleep phase disorder, free-running disorder, and irregular sleep-wake rhythm. An American Academy of Sleep Medicine review. Sleep 2007;30(11):1484–501.
3. Moore-Ede MC, Czeisler CA, Richardson GS. Circadian time-keeping in health and disease. I. Basic properties of circadian pacemakers. N Engl J Med 1983;309:469–76.
4. Wever RA. The circadian system of man. In: Topics in environmental physiology and medicine. New York: Springer-Verlag; 1979.
5. Okawa M, Uchiyama M. Circadian rhythm sleep disorders: characteristics and entrainment pathology in delayed sleep phase and non-24-h sleep-wake syndrome. Sleep Med Rev 2007;11(6):485–96.
6. Hayakawa T, Uchiyama M, Kamei Y, et al. Clinical analyses of sighted patients with non-24-h sleep–wake syndrome: a study of 57 consecutively diagnosed cases. Sleep 2005;28:945–52.
7. Lockley SW, Arendt J, Skene DJ. Visual impairment and circadian rhythm disorders. Dialogues Clin Neurosci 2007;9(3):301–14.

8. Flynn-Evans EE, Tabandeh H, Skene DJ, et al. Circadian rhythm disorders and melatonin production in 127 blind women with and without light perception. J Biol Rhythms 2014;29(3):215–24.

9. Uchiyama M, Okawa M, Ozaki S, et al. Delayed phase jumps of sleep onset in a patient with non-24-hour sleep-wake syndrome. Sleep 1996;19: 637–40.

10. Kokkoris CP, Weitzman ED, Pollak CP, et al. Long-term ambulatory temperature monitoring in a subject with a hypernychthemeral sleep-wake cycle disturbance. Sleep 1978;1:177–90.

11. Weber AL, Cary MS, Connor N, et al. Human non-24-hour sleep-wake cycles in an everyday environment. Sleep 1980;2:347–54.

12. Kamgar-Parsi B, Wehr TA, Gillin JC. Successful treatment of human non-24-hour sleep-wake syndrome. Sleep 1983;6:257–64.

13. Wollman M, Lavie P. Hypernychthemeral sleep-wake cycle: some hidden regularities. Sleep 1986;9:324–34.

14. Hoban TM, Sack RL, Lewy AJ, et al. Entrainment of a free-running human with bright light? Chronobiol Int 1989;6:347–53.

15. Okawa M, Uchiyama M, Shirakawa S, et al. Favourable effects of combined treatment with vitamin B12 and bright light for sleep-wake rhythm disorders. In: Kumar VM, Mallick HN, Nayar U, editors. Sleep-wakefulness. New Delhi (India): Wiley Eastern Ltd; 1993. p. 71–7.

16. Eliott AL, Mills JN, Waterhouse JM. A man with too long a day. J Physiol 1970;212:30–1.

17. Sugita Y, Ishikawa H, Mikami A, et al. Successful treatment for a patient with hypernychthemeral syndrome. Sleep Res 1987;16:642.

18. Eastman CI, Anagnopoulos CA, Cartwright RD. Can bright light entrain a free-runner? Sleep Res 1988;17:372.

19. Moriya Y, Yamazaki J, Higuchi T, et al. A case of non-24-hour sleep-wake syndrome. Jpn J Psychiatry Neurol 1990;44:189–90.

20. Sasaki T, Hashimoto O, Honda Y. A case of non-24-hour sleep-wake syndrome preceded by depressive state. Jpn J Psychiatry Neurol 1990; 44:191–2.

21. Ohta T, Ando K, Iwata T, et al. Treatment of persistent sleep-wake schedule disorders in adolescents with methylcobalamin (vitamin B12). Sleep 1991; 14:414–8.

22. Oren DA, Wehr TA. Hypernyctohemeral syndrome after chronotherapy for delayed sleep phase syndrome. N Engl J Med 1992;327:1762.

23. Tagaya H, Matsuno Y, Atsumi Y. A schizophrenic with non-24-hour sleep-wake syndrome. Jpn J Psychiatry Neurol 1993;47:441–2.

24. Emens JS, Brotman DJ, Czeisler CA. Evaluation of the intrinsic period of the circadian pacemaker in a patient with a non-24-hour sleep-wake schedule disorder. Sleep Res 1994;23:256.

25. Tomoda A, Miike T, Uezono K, et al. A school refusal case with biological rhythm disturbance and melatonin therapy. Brain Dev 1994;16:71–6.

26. McArthur AJ, Lewy AJ, Sack RL. Non-24-hour sleep-wake syndrome in a sighted man: circadian rhythm studies and efficacy of melatonin treatment. Sleep 1996;19:544–53.

27. Yamadera H, Takahashi K, Okawa M. A multicenter study of sleep-wake rhythm disorders: clinical features of sleep-wake rhythm disorders. Psychiatry Clin Neurosci 1996;50:195–201.

28. Nakamura K, Hashimoto S, Honma S, et al. A sighted man with non-24-hour sleep-wake syndrome shows damped plasma melatonin rhythm. Psychiatry Clin Neurosci 1997;51:115–9.

29. Shibui K, Uchiyama M, Iwama H, et al. Periodic fatigue symptoms due to desynchronization in a patient with non-24-hours sleep-wake syndrome. Psychiatry Clin Neurosci 1998;52:477–81.

30. Hashimoto S, Nakamura K, Honma S, et al. Free-running of plasma melatonin rhythm prior to full manifestation of a non-24 hour sleep-wake syndrome. Psychiatry Clin Neurosci 1998;52:264–5.

31. Hayakawa T, Kamei Y, Urata J, et al. Trials of bright light exposure and melatonin administration in a patient with non-24 hour sleep-wake syndrome. Psychiatry Clin Neurosci 1998;52:261–2.

32. Akaboshi S, Inoue Y, Kubota N, et al. Case of a mentally retarded child with non-24 hour sleep-wake syndrome caused by deficiency of melatonin secretion. Psychiatry Clin Neurosci 2000;54:379–80.

33. Watanabe T, Kajimura N, Kato M, et al. Case of a non-24 hours sleep-wake syndrome patient improved by phototherapy. Psychiatry Clin Neurosci 2000;54:369–70.

34. Morinobu S, Yamashita H, Yamawaki S, et al. Obsessive-compulsive disorder with non-24-hour sleep-wake syndrome. J Clin Psychiatry 2002;63:838–40.

35. Boivin DB, James FO, Santo JB, et al. Non-24-hour sleep-wake syndrome following a car accident. Neurology 2003;60:1841–3.

36. Dijk DJ, Czeisler CA. Contribution of the circadian pacemaker and the sleep homeostat to sleep propensity, sleep structure, electroencephalographic slow waves, and sleep spindle activity in humans. J Neurosci 1995;15(5 Pt 1):3526–38.

37. Boivin DB, Caliyurt O, James FO, et al. Association between delayed sleep phase and hypernyctohemeral syndromes: a case study. Sleep 2004; 27(3):417–21.

38. Crowley SJ, Acebo C, Carskadon MA. Sleep, circadian rhythms, and delayed phase in adolescence. Sleep Med 2007;8(6):602–12.

39. Uchiyama M, Okawa M, Shibui K, et al. Altered phase relation between sleep timing and core

body temperature rhythm in delayed sleep phase syndrome and non-24-h sleep–wake syndrome in humans. Neurosci Lett 2000;294:101–4.

40. Uchiyama M, Shibui K, Hayakawa T, et al. Larger phase angle between sleep propensity and melatonin rhythms in sighted humans with non-24-hour sleep-wake syndrome. Sleep 2002; 25:83–8.

41. Wulff K, Joyce E, Middleton B, et al. The suitability of actigraphy, diary data, and urinary melatonin profiles for quantitative assessment of sleep disturbances in schizophrenia: a case report. Chronobiol Int 2006;23(1–2):485–95.

42. Thorpy MJ, Korman E, Spielman AJ, et al. Delayed sleep phase syndrome in adolescents. J Adolesc Health Care 1988;9:22–7.

43. Regestein QR, Monk TH. Delayed sleep phase syndrome: a review of its clinical aspects. Am J Psychiatry 1995;152:602–8.

44. Wyatt JK. Delayed sleep phase syndrome: pathophysiology and treatment options. Sleep 2004; 27(6):1195–203.

45. Wehr TA, Wirz-Justice A, Goodwin FK, et al. Phase advance of the circadian sleep-wake cycle as an antidepressant. Science 1979;206:710–3.

46. Lewy AJ, Lefler BJ, Emens JS, et al. The circadian basis of winter depression. Proc Natl Acad Sci U S A 2006;103(19):7414–9.

47. Boivin DB. Influence of sleep-wake and circadian rhythm disturbances in psychiatric disorders. J Psychiatry Neurosci 2000;25(5):446–58.

48. Boivin DB, Czeisler CA, Dijk DJ, et al. Complex interaction of the sleep-wake cycle and circadian phase modulates mood in healthy subjects. Arch Gen Psychiatry 1997;54(2):145–52.

49. Surridge DM, MacLean A, Coulter ME, et al. Mood change following an acute delay of sleep. Psychiatry Res 1987;22:149–58.

50. Sack RL, Lewy AJ, Blood ML, et al. Circadian rhythm abnormalities in totally blind people: incidence and clinical significance. J Clin Endocrinol Metab 1992;75:127–34.

51. Lockley SW, Skene DJ, Arendt J, et al. Relationship between melatonin rhythms and visual loss in the blind. J Clin Endocrinol Metab 1997;82: 3763–70.

52. Skene DJ, Lockley SW, Thapan K, et al. Effects of light on human circadian rhythms. Reprod Nutr Dev 1999;39:295–304.

53. Lockley SW, Skene DJ, Butler LJ, et al. Sleep and activity rhythms are related to circadian phase in the blind. Sleep 1999;22(5):616–23.

54. Klerman EB, Rimmer DW, Dijk DJ, et al. Nonphotic entrainment of the human circadian pacemaker. Am J Physiol 1998;274(4 Pt 2):R991–6.

55. Mistlberger RE, Skene DJ. Nonphotic entrainment in humans? J Biol Rhythms 2005;20(4):339–52.

56. Czeisler CA, Shanahan TL, Klerman EB, et al. Suppression of melatonin secretion in some blind patients by exposure to bright light. N Engl J Med 1995;332(1):6–11.

57. Klerman EB, Shanahan TL, Brotman DJ, et al. Photic resetting of the human circadian pacemaker in the absence of conscious vision. J Biol Rhythms 2002;17(6):548–55.

58. Zaidi FH, Hull JT, Peirson SN, et al. Short-wavelength light sensitivity of circadian, pupillary, and visual awareness in humans lacking an outer retina. Curr Biol 2007;17(24):2122–8.

59. Gooley JJ, Ho Mien I, St Hilaire MA, et al. Melanopsin and rod-cone photoreceptors play different roles in mediating pupillary light responses during exposure to continuous light in humans. J Neurosci 2012;32(41):14242–53.

60. Vandewalle G, Collignon O, Hull JT, et al. Blue light stimulates cognitive brain activity in visually blind individuals. J Cogn Neurosci 2013;25(12):2072–85.

61. Leger D, Guilleminault C, Santos C, et al. Sleep/wake cycles in the dark: sleep recorded by polysomnography in 26 totally blind subjects compared to controls. Clin Neurophysiol 2002;113(10):1607–14.

62. Duffy JF, Cain SW, Chang AM, et al. Sex difference in the near-24-hour intrinsic period of the human circadian timing system. Proc Natl Acad Sci U S A 2011;108(Suppl 3):15602–8.

63. Emens JS, Laurie AL, Songer JB, et al. Non-24-Hour Disorder in blind individuals revisited: variability and the influence of environmental time cues. Sleep 2013;36(7):1091–100.

64. Eastman CI, Molina TA, Dziepak ME, et al. Blacks (African Americans) have shorter free-running circadian periods than whites (Caucasian Americans). Chronobiol Int 2012;29(8):1072–7.

65. Okawa M, Nanami T, Wada S, et al. Four congenitally blind children with circadian sleep–wake rhythm disorder. Sleep 1987;10:101–10.

66. Wee R, Van Gelder RN. Sleep disturbances in young subjects with visual dysfunction. Ophthalmology 2004;111(2):297–302.

67. Brainard GC, Hanifin JP. Photons, clocks, and consciousness. J Biol Rhythms 2005;20(4):314–25.

68. Peirson S, Foster RG. Melanopsin: another way of signaling light. Neuron 2006;49(3):331–9.

69. Lockley SW, Dijk DJ, Kosti O, et al. Alertness, mood and performance rhythm disturbances associated with circadian sleep disorders in the blind. J Sleep Res 2008;17(2):207–16.

70. Licamele L, Dressman M, Feeney J, et al. Pleiomorphic expression of Non-24-Hour disorder in the totally blind. Abstract. 13th meeting of the Society for Research in Biological Rhythms (SRBR). Destin, FL. May 19–23, 2012.

71. Klein T, Martens H, Dijk DJ, et al. Circadian sleep regulation in the absence of light perception:

chronic non-24-hour circadian rhythm sleep disorder in a blind man with a regular 24-hour sleep-wake schedule. Sleep 1993;16(4):333–43.

72. Czeisler CA, Weitzman ED, Moore-Ede MC, et al. Human sleep: its duration and organization depend on its circadian phase. Science 1980; 210:1264–7.

73. Sack RL, Brandes RW, Kendall AR, et al. Entrainment of free-running circadian rhythms by melatonin in blind people. N Engl J Med 2000;343(15):1070–7.

74. Miles LE, Raynal DM, Wilson MA. Blind man living in normal society has circadian rhythms of 24.9 hours. Science 1977;198(4315):421–3.

75. Lockley SW, Skene DJ, Arendt J. Comparison between subjective and actigraphic measurement of sleep and sleep rhythms. J Sleep Res 1999;8(3): 175–83.

76. Lewy AJ, Newsome DA. Different types of melatonin circadian secretory rhythms in some blind subjects. J Clin Endocrinol Metab 1983;56:1103–7.

77. Tabandeh H, Lockley SW, Buttery R, et al. Disturbance of sleep in blindness. Am J Ophthamol 1998;126:707–12.

78. Leger D, Guilleminault C, Defrance R, et al. Prevalence of sleep/wake disorders in persons with blindness. Clin Sci 1999;97:193–9.

79. Moseley MJ, Fouladi M, Jones HS, et al. Sleep disturbance and blindness. Lancet 1996; 348(9040):1514–5.

80. Dijk DJ, Lockley SW. Integration of human sleep-wake regulation and circadian rhythmicity. J Appl Physiol (1985) 2002;92(2):852–62.

81. Honma K, Honma S. A human phase response curve for bright light pulse. Jpn J Psychiatry Neurol 1988;42:167–8.

82. Minors DS, Waterhouse JM, Wirz-Justice A. A human phase–response curve to light. Neurosci Lett 1991;133:36–40.

83. Czeisler CA, Kronauer RE, Allan JS, et al. Bright light induction of strong (type 0) resetting of the human circadian pacemaker. Science 1989;244(4910): 1328–33.

84. St Hilaire MA, Gooley JJ, Khalsa SB, et al. Human phase response curve to a 1 h pulse of bright white light. J Physiol 2012;590(Pt 13):3035–45.

85. Czeisler CA, Duffy JF, Shanahan TL, et al. Stability, precision, and near-24-hour period of the human circadian pacemaker. Science 1999;284(5423): 2177–81.

86. Uchiyama M, Okawa M, Ozaki S, et al. Circadian characteristics of delayed sleep phase syndrome and non-24-hour sleep-wake syndrome. In: Honma K, Honma S, editors. Circadian clocks and entrainment. Sapporo (Japan): Hokkaido University Press; 1998. p. 115–30.

87. Uchiyama M, Okawa M, Shibui K, et al. Poor compensatory function for sleep loss as a pathologic factor in patients with delayed sleep phase syndrome. Sleep 2000;23:553–8.

88. Kitamura S, Hida A, Enomoto M, et al. Intrinsic circadian period of sighted patients with circadian rhythm sleep disorder, free-running type. Biol Psychiatry 2013;73(1):63–9.

89. Ralph MR, Meneker M. A mutation of the circadian system in golden hamster. Science 1988;241: 1225–7.

90. Vitaterna MH, King DP, Chang A, et al. Mutagenesis and mapping of a mouse gene, clock, essential for circadian behavior. Science 1994;264:719–21.

91. Ebisawa T. Circadian rhythms in the CNS and peripheral clock disorders: human sleep disorders and clock genes. J Pharmacol Sci 2007;103(2):150–4.

92. Jones CR, Campbell SS, Zone SE, et al. Familial advanced sleep-phase syndrome: a short-period circadian rhythm variant in humans. Nat Med 1999;5(9):1062–5.

93. Hida A, Kitamura S, Katayose Y, et al. Screening of clock gene polymorphisms demonstrates association of a PER3 polymorphism with morningness-eveningness preference and circadian rhythm sleep disorder. Sci Rep 2014;4:6309.

94. Kripke DF, Klimecki WT, Nievergelt CM, et al. Circadian polymorphisms in night owls, in bipolars, and in non-24-hour sleep cycles. Psychiatry Investig 2014;11(4):345–62.

95. Wright KP Jr, Drake CL, Lockley SW. Diagnostic tools for circadian rhythm sleep disorders. In: Kushida CA, editor. Handbook of sleep disorders. New York: Taylor & Francis Group, LLC; 2008. p. 147–73.

96. Benloucif S, Burgess HJ, Klerman EB, et al. Measuring melatonin in humans. J Clin Sleep Med 2008;4(1):66–9.

97. Lockley SW, Skene DJ, James K, et al. Melatonin administration can entrain the free-running circadian system of blind subjects. J Endocrinol 2000; 164:R1–6.

98. Lewy AJ, Ahmed S, Jackson JM, et al. Melatonin shifts human circadian rhythms according to a phase-response curve. Chronobiol Int 1992;9: 380–92.

99. Cajochen C, Kräuchi K, Wirz-Justice A. The acute soporific action of daytime melatonin administration: effects on the EEG during wakefulness and subjective alertness. J Biol Rhythms 1997;12(6): 636–43.

100. Kamei Y, Hayakawa T, Urata J, et al. Melatonin treatment for circadian rhythm sleep disorders. Psychiatry Clin Neurosci 2000;54:381–2.

101. Arendt J, Skene DJ, Middleton B, et al. Efficacy of melatonin treatment in jet lag, shift work, and blindness. J Biol Rhythms 1997;12(6):604–17.

102. Hack LM, Lockley SW, Arendt J, et al. The effects of low-dose 0.5-mg melatonin on the free-running

circadian rhythms of blind subjects. J Biol Rhythms 2003;18(5):420–9.

103. Lewy AJ, Bauer VK, Hasler BP, et al. Capturing the circadian rhythms of free-running blind people with 0.5 mg melatonin. Brain Res 2001;918:96–100.

104. Roth T, Nir T, Zisapel N. Prolonged release melatonin for improving sleep in totally blind subjects: a pilot placebo-controlled multicenter trial. Nat Sci Sleep 2015;7:13–23.

105. Lewy AJ, Emens JS, Sack RL, et al. Zeitgeber hierarchy in humans: resetting the circadian phase positions of blind people using melatonin. Chronobiol Int 2003;20:837–52.

106. Lewy AJ, Emens JS, Lefler BJ, et al. Melatonin entrains free-running blind people according to a physiological dose-response curve. Chronobiol Int 2005;22(6):1093–106.

107. Lewy AJ, Emens JS, Bernert RA, et al. Eventual entrainment of the human circadian pacemaker by melatonin is independent of the circadian phase of treatment initiation: clinical implications. J Biol Rhythms 2004;19(1):68–75.

108. Lewy AJ, Hasler BP, Emens JS, et al. Pretreatment circadian period in free-running blind people may predict the phase angle of entrainment to melatonin. Neurosci Lett 2001;313:158–60.

109. Arendt J. Safety of melatonin in long-term use (?). J Biol Rhythms 1997;12(6):673–81.

110. Buscemi N, Vandermeer B, Hooton N, et al. Efficacy and safety of exogenous melatonin for secondary sleep disorders and sleep disorders accompanying sleep restriction: meta-analysis. BMJ 2006;332(7538):385–93.

111. Rajaratnam SM, Polymeropoulos MH, Fisher DM, et al. Melatonin agonist tasimelteon (VEC-162) for transient insomnia after sleep-time shift: two randomised controlled multicentre trials. Lancet 2009; 373(9662):482–91 [Erratum appears in Lancet 2009;373(9671):1252].

112. Lavedan C, Forsberg M, Gentile AJ. Tasimelteon: a selective and unique receptor binding profile. Neuropharmacology 2015;91:142–7.

113. Lockley SW, Dressman MA, Licamele L, et al. Tasimelteon for non-24-hour sleep–wake disorder in totally blind people (SET and RESET): two multicentre, randomised, double-masked, placebo-controlled phase 3 trials. Lancet, in press. http://dx.doi.org/10.1016/S0140-6736(15)60031-9.

114. Yanagihara M, Nakamura M, Usui A, et al. The melatonin receptor agonist is effective for free-running type circadian rhythm sleep disorder: case report on two sighted patients. Tohoku J Exp Med 2014;234(2):123–8.

115. Yamadera H, Takahashi K, Okawa M. A multicenter study of sleep-wake rhythm disorders: therapeutic effects of vitamin B12, bright light therapy, chronotherapy and hypnotics. Psychiatry Clin Neurosci 1996;50(4):203–9.

116. Lee D, Shin WC. Forced entrainment by using light therapy, modafinil and melatonin in a sighted patient with non-24-hour sleep-wake disorder. Sleep Med 2015;16(2):305–7.

117. Sack RL, Lewy AJ, Hoban TM. Free-running melatonin rhythms in blind people: phase shifts with melatonin and triazolam administration. In: Rensing L, Van der Heiden U, Mackey MC, editors. Temporal disorder in human oscillatory systems. Heidelberg (Germany): Springer - Verlag; 1987. p. 219–24.

118. St Hilaire MA, Lockley SW. Caffeine does not entrain the circadian clock but improves daytime alertness in blind patients with non-24-hour rhythms. Sleep Med 2015;16(6):800–4.

Irregular Sleep-Wake Rhythm Disorder

Sabra M. Abbott, MD, PhD*, Phyllis C. Zee, MD, PhD

KEYWORDS

- Circadian rhythm • Suprachiasmatic nucleus • Sleep-wake rhythm disorder • Melatonin

KEY POINTS

- Irregular sleep-wake rhythm disorder (ISWRD) is a circadian rhythm disorder in which there is no clear sleep-wake pattern present.
- ISWRD is most commonly seen in children with neurodevelopmental delays and adults with neurodegenerative disease.
- Treatments are aimed at normalizing the day-night schedule, and increasing circadian amplitude by using a combination of melatonin, light, and sleep hygiene.

INTRODUCTION: NATURE OF THE PROBLEM

Individuals normally exhibit a near 24-hour or circadian pattern of behaviors and physiology, regulated by the central circadian pacemaker located in the suprachiasmatic nucleus (SCN). Irregular sleep-wake rhythm disorder (ISWRD) is a circadian rhythm disorder where there is no longer a clear 24-hour sleep-wake pattern. Individuals present with symptoms of either insomnia, excessive daytime sleepiness, or both, related to being awake during traditional sleep periods, and napping during the daytime.[1] The diagnosis of ISWRD depends on obtaining sleep-logs and/or actigraphy recordings from the individual for at least 1 but preferably 2 weeks. Sleep logs generally need to be completed by a caretaker given the high prevalence of neurologic impairment associated with this disorder. Actigraphy and sleep logs demonstrate at least three distinct sleep episodes within a 24-hour period; however, the total sleep for the entire day should be within normal limits for age (**Fig. 1**).[2,3] Usually sleep patterns consist of a slightly longer bout of sleep at night, with multiple naps throughout the day.

There are many factors that likely contribute to the development of ISWRD. There can be dysfunction at the level of the central pacemaker, the SCN, resulting in difficulty maintaining a 24-hour rhythm. There can also be pathology at the level of input to the SCN, either through impaired light pathways caused by retinal or optic nerve dysfunction, or through abnormal melatonin secretion. Finally, alterations in the social environment, with a lack of a clear day-night pattern, as can often be encountered in the nursing home or institutional environment can also contribute to development of this disorder. Just as the potential pathology of ISWRD is multifactorial, the populations that are affected by it are also quite diverse. Affected individuals can range from children with neurodevelopmental disorders to adults with neurodegenerative disease. An irregular sleep-wake rhythm can also be seen in some psychiatric disorders, with schizophrenia being the most frequently described. This disorder can result in significant negative consequences, particularly for caregivers who experience significant disruption to their own sleep as a result of the patient's inability to sleep through the night.

Disclosures: Dr S.M. Abbott has nothing to disclose. Dr P.C. Zee has served as a consultant for Vanda, Philips, Merck, and owns stock in Teva.
Department of Neurology, Northwestern Feinberg School of Medicine, 710 North Lake Shore Drive, Chicago, IL 60611, USA
* Corresponding author.
E-mail address: sabra.abbott@northwestern.edu

Sleep Med Clin 10 (2015) 517–522
http://dx.doi.org/10.1016/j.jsmc.2015.08.005

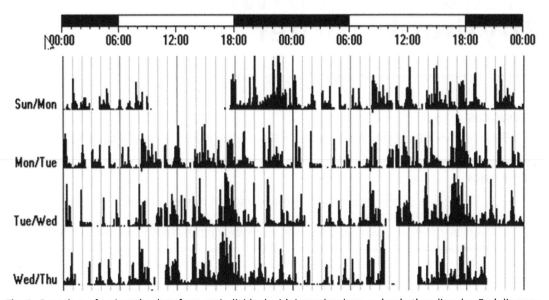

Fig. 1. Four days of actigraphy data from an individual with irregular sleep-wake rhythm disorder. Each line represents 48 hours, with the last 24 hours of each line replotted on the following line. Vertical black lines indicate activity. There is no clear rest activity pattern noted.

Many neurodevelopmental disorders in children have been associated with ISWRD. In a case series of four congenitally blind, neurodevelopmentally delayed children, most exhibited a non-24-hour or free-running pattern; however, one exhibited an irregular rest activity pattern, suggesting impairment of light input to the SCN and a primary impairment at the level of the circadian pacemaker.[4] Patients with neuronal ceroid-lipofuscinosis, a neurodegenerative disorder associated with impaired cognition and optic atrophy and retinal degeneration, frequently exhibit an irregular sleep-wake pattern. However, despite abnormal rest activity patterns, the daily rhythms of melatonin and cortisol do not seem to be significantly disrupted in these individuals, only becoming disrupted late in the course of the illness. In addition, core body temperature rhythms were only disrupted in approximately half of the children studied, suggesting the primary pathology may stem from the lack of visual input secondary to the optic atrophy and retinal degeneration.[5]

In patients with Angelman syndrome, a neurodevelopmental disorder characterized by mental retardation, seizures, gait and speech impairment, epilepsy, and craniofacial abnormalities, circadian rhythm sleep-wake disorders are common. ISWRD occurs most frequently, but delayed sleep-wake phase disorder and non-24-hour sleep-wake rhythm disorder have also been observed. These individuals have also been noted to have a decrease in nocturnal melatonin levels corresponding with their sleep-wake disturbances.[6]

Smith-Magenis syndrome is a genetic disorder characterized by behavioral problems, craniofacial abnormalities, and sleep disturbances, thought to be related to abnormal melatonin secretion patterns. Although the most common sleep disturbance observed is a complete inversion of the sleep-wake schedule, these individuals also occasionally present with ISWRD.[7] Finally, children with autism spectrum disorder have also been demonstrated to have an irregular sleep-wake pattern, thought in part to be caused by an increased sensitivity to external noise resulting in greater sleep fragmentation.[8]

In a case series of elderly patients with dementia, caretaker assessments of the sleep-wake pattern demonstrated either inverted or irregular sleep-wake patterns in most individuals, with an overall decrease in the amplitude of the rest-activity rhythm. In addition, this decreased amplitude corresponded with abnormal patterns of the core body temperature rhythm.[9] Later studies have demonstrated similar findings with wrist actigraphy monitoring, demonstrating decreased overall activity, decreased circadian amplitude, and increased fragmentation of the rest-activity rhythm in patients with dementia.[10] Interestingly, the magnitude of decreased rest-activity amplitude correlates with the severity of dementia.[10] Also, increased fragmentation of the rest-activity pattern correlates with greater impairment in cognitive performance.[11]

Both aging and Alzheimer disease (AD) have also been associated with a decrease in amplitude of the daily melatonin rhythm.[12,13] The observed sleep and circadian abnormalities are thought to be caused by several factors, including decreased visual input to the SCN, lack of a strong day-night rhythm in the institutionalized environment, and alterations in neuronal function at the level of the SCN. In evidence supporting this theory, it has been demonstrated that in patients with AD a decrease in the amplitude of the rest-activity rhythm correlated with a decrease in number of cells in the SCN.[14] In addition, postmortem analysis of brain tissue from patients with AD has demonstrated that circadian clock gene expression patterns are no longer synchronized throughout the brain, again suggesting pathology in the underlying clock mechanisms.[15] There is also evidence that the observed sleep abnormalities may actually precede the onset of dementia, and may be either an early symptom of the disease or part of the underlying pathology, rather than just a result of underlying illness. In a large study evaluating actigraphy in more than 1200 healthy women, decreased amplitude and robustness of the circadian rhythm of rest-activity was associated with an increased risk for the development of either mild cognitive impairment or dementia over the next 5 years.[16]

ISWRD can also be seen in psychiatric disorders. Several studies have evaluated rest activity patterns in schizophrenia, and have demonstrated an irregular sleep-wake pattern in a significant number of patients.[17-19] ISWRD is more common in patients with predominantly positive symptoms,[17] and has also been associated with decreased cognitive performance.[18] Nocturnal plasma melatonin levels have also been demonstrated to be lower in patients with schizophrenia, resulting in an overall decrease in the 24-hour amplitude of the melatonin rhythm.[20]

Finally, ISWRD can also result from pathologic disruption of the SCN and the sleep-wake regulatory pathways, either through trauma or malignant pathology. Traumatic brain injury is frequently associated with sleep disturbance, with a high incidence of circadian rhythm sleep-wake disorders, including delayed sleep-wake phase disorder, non-24-hour sleep-wake rhythm disorder, and ISWRD. Traumatic brain injury patients with ISWRD often either have decreased amplitude or complete lack of a 24-hour rhythm of oral temperature.[21] The observed circadian abnormalities are thought to be caused by either disruption of the primary pacemaker and/or the pathways regulating the daily pattern of melatonin release. In support of this, one case report demonstrated development of ISWRD following a gunshot injury resulting in damage to the SCN and bilateral optic nerves.[22] Sleep disturbances are also frequently reported in child and adult survivors of brain tumors, particularly those with craniopharyngiomas, which often impact the hypothalamus.[23] There is also a case report of ISWRD emerging following the development of a prolactin-secreting pituitary microadenoma that impinged on the SCN. This individual's rest-activity pattern was disrupted, and analysis of circadian biomarkers demonstrated a salivary melatonin period of 24 hours, but a core body temperature of 28 hours suggesting the irregular sleep-wake pattern developed secondary to internal desynchronization of the circadian clock.[24]

THERAPEUTIC OPTIONS AND OUTCOMES

Treatment of ISWRD depends on multiple interventions aimed at increasing the overall circadian amplitude and stabilizing the day-night rhythm. Interventions include timed melatonin and bright light administration, behavioral interventions to improve the overall circadian amplitude and consolidate the sleep-wake pattern, or a combination of all of these, as outlined in **Table 1**.

Melatonin administered at bedtime is frequently used as a treatment of ISWRD, although in children there are no randomized controlled trials demonstrating the effectiveness of this intervention. In a group of five children with severe psychomotor retardation and a decreased amplitude of melatonin secretion, administration of 3 mg of melatonin in the evening resulted in an increase in nocturnal sleep by 1.4 hours, and a decrease in daytime sleep by 1.5 hours, without significantly changing the 24-hour total sleep time.[25] Administration of 1 mg of melatonin between 6 and 7 PM in patients with Angelman syndrome and ISWRD resulted in a significant increase in the percentage of sleep occurring at night compared with during the day.[6] In a larger open-label trial, doses of melatonin ranging from 2 to 20 mg have been demonstrated to be effective at normalizing sleep-wake patterns in children with neurodevelopmental delay.[26] In patients with schizophrenia, a small randomized controlled trial demonstrated improvement in actigraphically measured sleep following administration of melatonin (2 mg) at bedtime.[27] However, in adults with dementia, two separate randomized placebo-controlled trials failed to demonstrate a benefit in actigraphically measured sleep with the use of melatonin alone.[28,29]

Bright light exposure in patients with AD has been shown to be beneficial regardless of whether it is administered in the morning or evening. Morning bright light (>2500 lux) has been shown to increase nighttime sleep by 20 to 30 minutes,

Table 1
Current evidence for treatment options for irregular sleep-wake rhythm disorder in different populations

Treatment	Population	Current Data
Light	Children (with intact visual input to the SCN)	Morning bright light (4500 lux) normalized the sleep-wake cycle (in some children).[33]
	Adults with dementia	Daytime bright light exposure (2500 lux) may increase total sleep time at night.[30]
Melatonin	Children	Doses ranging from 2 to 20 mg have been shown to normalize sleep-wake patterns.[26,29]
	Adults with dementia	Randomized controlled trials have not demonstrated an improvement in actigraphically measured sleep.[28] Caution when using alone, without light, because can worsen mood.[31]
	Schizophrenia	In a randomized controlled trial, 2 mg of melatonin at bedtime improved actigraphically measured sleep.[27]
Mixed-modality treatment	Adults with dementia	Morning bright light (>10,000 lux), low-level physical activity, structured bedtime routine, and efforts to minimize light and noise at night.[35,36]

whereas evening bright light exposure has been demonstrated to improve the consolidation of the rest-activity rhythm.[30] Continuous daytime bright light exposure (1000 lux) has been associated with an increased total sleep time, improved inter-daily stability of the rest activity rhythm, and improved overall mood.[31] More recently a study designed to develop a more practical intervention installed tailored room lighting to provide increased bright light exposure during the day, whenever the subject was in their room, to improve compliance with the intervention by eliminating the need to position the patients in front of light boxes for set time periods. Under these conditions, total sleep time and sleep efficiency increased and there was an increase in overall circadian entrainment when evaluating the rest-activity pattern in relation to the light exposure.[32] Similarly, in a small population of children with neurodevelopmental delay, morning bright light (4500 lux) resulted in normalization of sleep-wake patterns in approximately half of the children studied.[33]

Of note, the use of light depends on having intact light input pathways to the SCN, which can often be impaired in individuals with ISWRD. In at least one child with congenital blindness and neurodevelopmental delay, the only treatment that was effective at normalizing her sleep-wake schedule was a focus on strong social cues, presumably because of an absence of light-entraining mechanisms and of a functioning central pacemaker.[4] Similarly

behavioral interventions with strong social cues were the only interventions found to be effective for the woman with a gunshot injury resulting in trauma to the SCN and bilateral optic nerves.[22] However, even in individuals with intact retinal inputs to the SCN, this strategy can be effective, as demonstrated in a population of individuals with dementia, where increasing social interaction during the day resulted in improvements of the sleep-wake rhythm, although the associated abnormal core body temperature rhythm did not show corresponding improvements.[9]

Daytime sleep, nocturnal sleep disturbances, and an overall irregular sleep-wake pattern are extremely common among nursing home residents. Part of the problem seems to stem from patients spending large amounts of time during the day in their rooms, in bed, with minimal social activity during the day to keep them awake and active in conjunction with increased noise and sleep disruption at night.[34] To modify these behaviors and improve overall sleep quality in these individuals a strategy termed "mixed modality treatment" was developed. This consists of a combination of efforts to keep subjects out of bed during the day, low level daytime physical activity, at least 30 minutes of morning bright light exposure (>10,000 lux), a structured bedtime routine, and efforts to minimize light and noise at night. This combination of therapies resulted in a significant decrease in daytime sleep, and a small improvement in nighttime sleep in two separate populations of elderly individuals with dementia.[35,36]

COMPLICATIONS AND CONCERNS

An alternative, although not recommended, strategy that is often used in the treatment of these individuals is to use hypnotics to increase nocturnal sleep. However, the concern with this strategy is that the use of hypnotics may lead to a pseudonormalization of the sleep-wake pattern, without actually addressing the underlying circadian disorder. In addition, there is growing evidence that hypnotic use, particularly in the elderly, may be associated with an increased risk for delirium and falls. Both the benzodiazepine and nonbenzodiazepine hypnotics have recently been included in the American Geriatric Society's Beers criteria for potentially inappropriate medications for use in the elderly.[37]

Melatonin use alone can also occasionally be problematic in the elderly, with at least one study demonstrating that melatonin use alone (2.5 mg) in a population of elderly nursing home residents was associated with adverse effects on mood, although mood improved with the addition of bright light therapy.[31]

Although light therapy has generally been demonstrated to be beneficial in the elderly, at least one study has reported an increase in agitation in a population of demented individuals following exposure to morning, evening, or all-day light when compared with standard lighting conditions. Thus, close observation is recommended following any recommendations to initiate light therapy for patients.[38]

SUMMARY

Overall ISWRD can be debilitating for individuals affected by the disorder. However, unlike many of the other circadian rhythm sleep-wake disorders it also results in significant caretaker burden because of the inability of the patient to maintain a consolidated sleep-wake pattern and the high degree of neurologic impairment often seen in these individuals. Because the circadian dysfunction is often multifactorial, either resulting from a dysfunctional pacemaker, impaired input to the SCN either from the eye or pineal, or living in an environment with minimal daily activity and nocturnal sleep disruption, treatment strategies also need to focus on a multifactorial approach. However, current strategies still only have limited success, and with the growing number of individuals with dementia in the population, greater attention should be paid to finding more effective strategies for managing this disorder.

REFERENCES

1. ICSD-3. The International Classification of Sleep Disorders: diagnostic and coding manual. 2nd edition. Darien (IL): American Academy of Sleep Medicine; 2014.
2. Sack RL, Auckley D, Auger RR, et al. Circadian rhythm sleep disorders: part II, advanced sleep phase disorder, delayed sleep phase disorder, free-running disorder, and irregular sleep-wake rhythm. An American Academy of Sleep Medicine review. Sleep 2007;30(11):1484–501.
3. Zee PC, Vitiello MV. Circadian rhythm sleep disorder: irregular sleep wake rhythm type. Sleep Med Clin 2009;4(2):213–8.
4. Okawa M, Nanami T, Wada S, et al. Four congenitally blind children with circadian sleep-wake rhythm disorder. Sleep 1987;10(2):101–10.
5. Heikkila E, Hatonen TH, Telakivi T, et al. Circadian rhythm studies in neuronal ceroid-lipofuscinosis (NCL). Am J Med Genet 1995;57(2):229–34.
6. Takaesu Y, Komada Y, Inoue Y. Melatonin profile and its relation to circadian rhythm sleep disorders in Angelman syndrome patients. Sleep Med 2012;13(9):1164–70.
7. Potocki L, Glaze D, Tan DX, et al. Circadian rhythm abnormalities of melatonin in Smith-Magenis syndrome. J Med Genet 2000;37(6):428–33.
8. Cortesi F, Giannotti F, Ivanenko A, et al. Sleep in children with autistic spectrum disorder. Sleep Med 2010;11(7):659–64.
9. Okawa M, Mishima K, Hishikawa Y, et al. Circadian rhythm disorders in sleep-waking and body temperature in elderly patients with dementia and their treatment. Sleep 1991;14(6):478–85.
10. Witting W, Kwa IH, Eikelenboom P, et al. Alterations in the circadian rest-activity rhythm in aging and Alzheimer's disease. Biol Psychiatry 1990;27(6):563–72.
11. Lim AS, Yu L, Costa MD, et al. Increased fragmentation of rest-activity patterns is associated with a characteristic pattern of cognitive impairment in older individuals. Sleep 2012;35(5):633–640B.
12. Ohashi Y, Okamoto N, Uchida K, et al. Daily rhythm of serum melatonin levels and effect of light exposure in patients with dementia of the Alzheimer's type. Biol Psychiatry 1999;45(12):1646–52.
13. Skene DJ, Swaab DF. Melatonin rhythmicity: effect of age and Alzheimer's disease. Exp Gerontol 2003;38(1–2):199–206.
14. Wang JL, Lim AS, Chiang WY, et al. Suprachiasmatic neuron numbers and rest-activity circadian rhythms in older humans. Ann Neurol 2015;78(2):317–22.
15. Cermakian N, Lamont EW, Boudreau P, et al. Circadian clock gene expression in brain regions of Alzheimer's disease patients and control subjects. J Biol Rhythms 2011;26(2):160–70.
16. Tranah GJ, Blackwell T, Stone KL, et al. Circadian activity rhythms and risk of incident dementia and mild cognitive impairment in older women. Ann Neurol 2011;70(5):722–32.

17. Afonso P, Brissos S, Figueira ML, et al. Schizophrenia patients with predominantly positive symptoms have more disturbed sleep-wake cycles measured by actigraphy. Psychiatry Res 2011; 189(1):62–6.

18. Bromundt V, Koster M, Georgiev-Kill A, et al. Sleep-wake cycles and cognitive functioning in schizophrenia. Br J Psychiatry 2011;198(4):269–76.

19. Wulff K, Dijk DJ, Middleton B, et al. Sleep and circadian rhythm disruption in schizophrenia. Br J Psychiatry 2012;200(4):308–16.

20. Vigano D, Lissoni P, Rovelli F, et al. A study of light/dark rhythm of melatonin in relation to cortisol and prolactin secretion in schizophrenia. Neuro Endocrinol Lett 2001;22(2):137–41.

21. Ayalon L, Borodkin K, Dishon L, et al. Circadian rhythm sleep disorders following mild traumatic brain injury. Neurology 2007;68(14):1136–40.

22. DelRosso LM, Hoque R, James S, et al. Sleep-wake pattern following gunshot suprachiasmatic damage. J Clin Sleep Med 2014;10(4):443–5.

23. Gapstur R, Gross CR, Ness K. Factors associated with sleep-wake disturbances in child and adult survivors of pediatric brain tumors: a review. Oncol Nurs Forum 2009;36(6):723–31.

24. Borodkin K, Ayalon L, Kanety H, et al. Dysregulation of circadian rhythms following prolactin-secreting pituitary microadenoma. Chronobiol Int 2005;22(1):145–56.

25. Pillar G, Shahar E, Peled N, et al. Melatonin improves sleep-wake patterns in psychomotor retarded children. Pediatr Neurol 2000;23(3):225–8.

26. Jan JE, Espezel H, Appleton RE. The treatment of sleep disorders with melatonin. Dev Med Child Neurol 1994;36(2):97–107.

27. Shamir E, Laudon M, Barak Y, et al. Melatonin improves sleep quality of patients with chronic schizophrenia. J Clin Psychiatry 2000;61(5):373–7.

28. Serfaty M, Kennell-Webb S, Warner J, et al. Double blind randomised placebo controlled trial of low dose melatonin for sleep disorders in dementia. Int J Geriatr Psychiatry 2002;17(12):1120–7.

29. Singer C, Tractenberg RE, Kaye J, et al. A multicenter, placebo-controlled trial of melatonin for sleep disturbance in Alzheimer's disease. Sleep 2003;26(7):893–901.

30. Ancoli-Israel S, Gehrman P, Martin JL, et al. Increased light exposure consolidates sleep and strengthens circadian rhythms in severe Alzheimer's disease patients. Behav Sleep Med 2003;1(1):22–36.

31. Riemersma-van der Lek RF, Swaab DF, Twisk J, et al. Effect of bright light and melatonin on cognitive and noncognitive function in elderly residents of group care facilities: a randomized controlled trial. JAMA 2008;299(22):2642–55.

32. Figueiro MG, Plitnick BA, Lok A, et al. Tailored lighting intervention improves measures of sleep, depression, and agitation in persons with Alzheimer's disease and related dementia living in long-term care facilities. Clin Interv Aging 2014;9:1527–37.

33. Guilleminault C, McCann CC, Quera-Salva M, et al. Light therapy as treatment of dyschronosis in brain impaired children. Eur J Pediatr 1993;152(9):754–9.

34. Martin JL, Webber AP, Alam T, et al. Daytime sleeping, sleep disturbance, and circadian rhythms in the nursing home. Am J Geriatr Psychiatry 2006;14(2):121–9.

35. Alessi CA, Martin JL, Webber AP, et al. Randomized, controlled trial of a nonpharmacological intervention to improve abnormal sleep/wake patterns in nursing home residents. J Am Geriatr Soc 2005;53(5):803–10.

36. McCurry SM, Gibbons LE, Logsdon RG, et al. Nighttime insomnia treatment and education for Alzheimer's disease: a randomized, controlled trial. J Am Geriatr Soc 2005;53(5):793–802.

37. American Geriatrics Society Beers Criteria Update Expert Panel. American Geriatrics Society updated Beers Criteria for potentially inappropriate medication use in older adults. J Am Geriatr Soc 2012; 60(4):616–31.

38. Barrick AL, Sloane PD, Williams CS, et al. Impact of ambient bright light on agitation in dementia. Int J Geriatr Psychiatry 2010;25(10):1013–21.

Jet Lag and Shift Work Disorder

Kathryn J. Reid, PhD[a],*, Sabra M. Abbott, MD, PhD[b]

KEYWORDS

- Irregular schedules • Transmeridian travel • Night work • Jet lag • Shift work • Sleep loss
- Circadian misalignment

KEY POINTS

- Severity of jet lag symptoms depends on direction of travel (east or west) and number of time zones crossed.
- Shift work disorder is characterized by insomnia and/or excessive sleepiness associated with the work schedule and associated with increased risk of obesity, diabetes, hypertension, depression, cognitive impairment, and cancer.
- Treatment of shift work disorder and jet lag disorder aim to realign the endogenous circadian clock with the required work schedule and/or environment.
- Studies are needed to determine the efficacy of treatments for jet lag and shift work disorder currently recommended by the American Academy of Sleep Medicine.
- Development and testing of interventions to improve long-term health outcomes for shift workers are needed.

INTRODUCTION

The circadian system regulates the timing of almost all of our physiologic functions, including blood pressure, core body temperature, hunger, mood, cognitive function, and hormonal profiles of cortisol and melatonin, as well as insulin sensitivity.[1] Circadian rhythms are controlled by a master pacemaker, the suprachiasmatic nucleus, which is located in the anterior hypothalamus.[2] However, we now know that almost all cells of the body have molecular clocks, so that all major organ systems including the heart, lungs, liver, and pancreas have their own distinct circadian timing.[3,4] All of these peripheral systems need to work in synchrony to maintain optimal health.

The circadian clock oscillates with a period that is typically slightly longer than 24 hours in humans.[5] Although circadian rhythms are generated endogenously, they are influenced strongly by the environmental light–dark cycle. In the absence of external time cues, the timing of circadian rhythms, including sleep and wake timing, will drift later each day.[6,7] When the timing of the light–dark cycle is altered as a result of transmeridian travel or shift work, it leads to misalignment of the circadian system with the external physical or work environment. Circadian misalignment has been shown to result in poor sleep and performance and on a more chronic basis is thought to lead to poor health outcomes, including obesity, hypertension, diabetes, and cancer.[8]

The 2 most common causes of circadian disruption in today's modern 24/7 society are jet lag and shift work. Although modern aircraft can travel

The authors have nothing to disclose.

[a] Department of Neurology, Center for Circadian and Sleep Medicine, Feinberg School of Medicine, Northwestern University, 710 North Lakeshore Drive, Room 522, Chicago, IL 60611, USA; [b] Department of Neurology, Center for Circadian and Sleep Medicine, Feinberg School of Medicine, Northwestern University, 710 North Lakeshore Drive, Room 524, Chicago, IL 60611, USA

* Corresponding author.

E-mail address: k-reid@northwestern.edu

Sleep Med Clin 10 (2015) 523–535

http://dx.doi.org/10.1016/j.jsmc.2015.08.006

across multiple time zones in just a few hours, the speed with which our circadian clock adjusts to these changes in the external environment takes much longer. For shift workers, the constant alternation between a conventional sleep–wake schedule and being awake at night and sleeping during the day not only alters the light–dark cycle in relation to the endogenous circadian clock, but also alters feeding patterns. For some people, this mismatch between the endogenous circadian clock and the external environment results in a circadian rhythm sleep–wake disorder that is typically characterized by symptoms of insomnia, excessive sleepiness, fatigue, and physical complaints, such as gastrointestinal disruption, that negatively impact daily functioning. The aim of this article is to describe the criteria for and diagnosis and treatment of 2 circadian rhythm sleep–wake disorders, namely, jet lag disorder and shift work disorder.[9,10]

GENERAL THERAPEUTIC APPROACHES

There are 2 general approaches to address the symptoms of jet lag and shift work disorder. The first is to accelerate realignment of the circadian system with the external environment and the second is to treat the symptoms of insomnia and excessive sleepiness. Multimodal approaches are typically needed and should be tailored to the individual, because the severity of symptoms and timing of treatments depends on the direction of travel and number of times zones crossed or the type of work schedule. For clarity, each disorder is discussed separately.

Phase shifting, or resetting the circadian clock, is achieved by timed light–dark exposure and or melatonin administration. The time of administration of these interventions determines whether they result in a phase delay (later) or phase advance (earlier). Light before the core body temperature minimum (T_{min}) results in a phase delay, whereas light after the T_{min} results in a phase advance.[11,12] The intensity, duration of exposure, and wavelength of light also influence the degree to which the circadian clock will phase shift.[11–16] The response for melatonin is opposite to light, with melatonin before the T_{min} resulting in a phase advance and melatonin after the T_{min} resulting in a phase delay.[17,18] The largest phase advances are achieved with low doses ($\leq$3 mg) of melatonin about 4 hours before habitual dim light melatonin onset, or 6 hours before habitual sleep onset.[19]

Most treatments for jet lag and shift work disorder are derived from small, single-center studies. There is a need for more large-scale, multicenter, placebo-controlled clinical trials to assess not only the efficacy, but also the real-world effectiveness of the currently available treatments, and for the development of improved behavioral and pharmacologic strategies. With this in mind, the therapeutic options described herein are the current standard of care based on the recommendations outlined by the American Academy of Sleep Medicine[20]; further research is still needed.

JET LAG DISORDER

Jet lag disorder results from rapidly crossing at least 2 times zones, with the severity of symptoms typically depending on both the number of times zones crossed and the direction of travel (east or west). Symptoms include insomnia, excessive sleepiness, and decreases in total sleep time.[9,10] There is limited information on the prevalence of jet lag, but given the increasing frequency of international airline travel it is suspected to be quite high.[21,22] Age may predispose people to suffer more symptoms of jet lag. There are various reasons patients seek treatment for jet lag disorder; however, primarily they do so when the symptoms are severe, whether the travel is for recreation or business. A summary of the symptoms, diagnosis, and treatment of jet lag disorder are provided in **Table 1**.

As mentioned, jet lag disorder can be treated by addressing directly the symptoms of insomnia and sleepiness, or by speeding the adjustment, or entrainment of the circadian clock to the new time zone. Although the treatment of symptoms is similar for both eastward and westward travel, approaches that address realigning the circadian system require administration of treatments at different times, depending on the direction of travel.

Practicing good sleep hygiene while traveling is a key approach to improve sleep and speed entrainment to the new environment. Therefore, patients should keep a regular sleep–wake schedule, and sleep in a dark, quiet, and cool environment whenever possible. Other general recommendations that may help to reduce the symptoms of jet lag are to avoid excessive alcohol or caffeine consumption, drink plenty of water to remain hydrated, sleep as much as possible on long flights, and eat meals at appropriate local times once arriving at the new destination. Caffeine and short naps either alone or in combination can be used to improve alertness during the day, but should be avoided close to bedtime.

For travelers who plan to be in the new time for just 1 or 2 days, symptomatic management with short-acting hypnotics (if an adequate sleep opportunity is available) and/or alertness-enhancing

Table 1
Summary of the symptoms, diagnosis, and treatment of shift work disorder

Symptoms	Diagnosis	Treatment
• Sleep initiation and maintenance insomnia and/or • Excessive sleepiness while at work	• Clinical history • Sleep log and/or wrist actigraphy monitoring for 2 wk	• Sleep hygiene • Scheduled light/dark exposure • Avoid bright light in the morning after night shift • Bright light or intermittent bright light (3000–10,000 lux) in the first half of the night shift • Scheduled naps (20–30 min) during work if allowed or longer before work to supplement main sleep period • Wake promoting agents - modafinil or armodafinil (FDA approved), caffeine (avoid close to sleep time) • Melatonin (1–3 mg) before the daytime sleep • Hypnotics

Abbreviation: FDA, US Food and Drug Administration.

medications might be preferred. Treatments that aim to realign the circadian clock to the new time zone are not recommended if travel to the new location is for 2 days or longer.[9,10] However, if the person has an important event for which peak performance is required, adjustment to the new time zone can be achieved by initiating circadian phase adjustment before travel.[23]

Traveling East

When traveling east, the circadian clock needs to phase advance, or move earlier. In general, it is more difficult for the circadian clock to phase advance than to phase delay, because the intrinsic period of the circadian clock in humans is on average longer than 24 hours,[5] and as such, symptoms of jet lag may persist for longer and be worse than for westward travel. Combining behavioral interventions, modified light–dark exposure, and melatonin or melatonin agonist administration is likely to be the most beneficial treatment strategy, although there are currently no field studies to support such a combination strategy in jet lag disorder. A schematic example of the timing of sleep–wake schedule circadian markers, and treatment options for eastward travel between Chicago and Brussels are provided in **Fig. 1**.

Treatment for jet lag disorder can begin before travel. Beginning to adjust the circadian clock to the new time zone before travel may be desirable for some travelers, especially if they want to be functioning at their best immediately upon arrival in the new time zone. Studies in the laboratory have shown that starting circadian interventions about 3 days before the day of travel, combining advancing the sleep schedule with appropriately timed bright light and melatonin administration can phase advance the circadian clock by about 2.5 hours and is also beneficial for sleep and well-being.[23] The patient would start by altering their sleep–wake schedule and go to bed an hour earlier each day. They would also aim to get approximately an hour of bright light (four 30-minute pulses of 5000 lux) in the morning, and to take low-dose melatonin (1–3 mg) 5 hours before their usual sleep time.[23,24] A limitation of this approach is that patients may not have the time or flexibility in their usual schedule to alter their sleep–wake schedule or to sit in front of a light box in the morning before travel. Because one of the challenges of light administration as a treatment is the time required sitting in front of a light box, a recent laboratory based study examined the effectiveness of 3 different light interventions (~5000 lux) combined with shifts in sleep–wake and melatonin administration similar to those described.[25] The largest phase shifts were achieved with four 30-minute exposures (2.4 hours), and similar shifts were achieved with four 15-minute exposures (1.7 hours), and a single 30-minute exposure (1.8 hours). The authors conclude that a single 30-minute exposure may be adequate to phase advance the circadian clock when in combination with altered sleep–wake and afternoon melatonin administration.

Treatment for jet lag disorder when the patient arrives in the new destination after eastward travel is as follows. In the new time zone, the light–dark

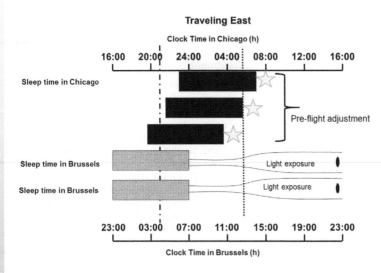

Traveling East

Clock Time in Chicago (h)

Sleep time in Chicago

Pre-flight adjustment

Sleep time in Brussels — Light exposure

Sleep time in Brussels — Light exposure

Clock Time in Brussels (h)

Fig. 1. Circadian rhythm sleep–wake disorder, jet lag disorder, and circadian-based treatment recommendations when traveling east from Chicago to Brussels. The black bar indicates the sleep period when in Chicago, white indicates wake, the hatched bars indicate the sleep period in Brussels, the line with dashes and dots indicates the approximate timing of the melatonin onset, and the dotted line indicates the core body temperature minimum (T_{min}). The recommended timing of light exposure is indicated by the black curved lines, the black ovals indicate exogenous melatonin administration. If circadian rhythms and the sleep–wake cycle are in phase, the melatonin onset would occur about 2 hours before sleep onset, and the T_{min} would occur about 2 hours before wake. Jet lag disorder occurs when traveling in an eastward direction because the sleep period is advanced in relation to the internal circadian clock, and because sleep is attempted before the melatonin onset there is difficulty falling asleep and because the rise time is before the T_{min}, there is sleepiness upon awakening. To treat this disorder a phase advance of the circadian clock is required. If attempting preflight adjustment, the recommendation if to start 3 days before travel and to shift the sleep period earlier each day by an hour and to get bright light in the morning (indicated by the *star*). Upon arrival in Brussels it is recommended to avoid light in the morning upon waking because this would be before the T_{min} (even with preflight adjustment) and light exposure at this circadian time would result in a phase delay. Melatonin taken at bedtime should also aid in the phase advance.

schedule will be shifted in relation to internal timing, and as such, managing light and dark exposure is important to maximize the realignment of the circadian clock to the new time zone.[26,27] At the new destination, the patient should avoid morning light by wearing sunglasses or remaining indoors, and seek afternoon bright light exposure by either going outside or by using a light box.[27,28] Melatonin can also be taken before bedtime (2–5 mg) both for its hypnotic effects and ability to phase shift the circadian clock.[29–32] Hypnotics can also be used before sleep. zolpidem (10 mg) has been studied in this context and shown to be useful.[32,33] Ramelteon, an MT1/MT2 melatonin receptor agonist taken before bedtime, has also been shown to improve sleep after a 5-hour phase advance after traveling east, with the 1-mg dose producing the greatest effect on latency to persistent sleep.[34]

Traveling West

For westward travel, approaches are similar to those for eastward travel; however, the goal is now to phase delay the circadian clock, so the timing of the entraining agents (light, activity, and melatonin) are at different times than for eastward travel.

If preflight adjustment is desired, there is a simulated laboratory study that indicates that a single day with a 4-hour delay of bedtime and 2 hours of bright light exposure (~4000 lux) before bed will phase delay the circadian clock by about 1.5 hours.[35] If a similar protocol is followed for 4 days, a phase delay of up to 4.4 hours can be achieved, in this longer study they used only a 2-hour delay of the sleep period, during which a bright light pulse of ~5000 lux was given.[36]

Once arriving at the new destination, the patient should avoid morning light and seek evening light. There are also 2 studies in jet travelers demonstrating that 5 mg of melatonin taken before departure (~10 AM to 12 PM) and upon arrival in the new destination (~10 PM to 12 AM) subjectively improves the symptoms of jet lag after westward travel.[37,38]

Other Treatment Considerations for Jet Lag Disorder

Symptoms of jet lag should dissipate once the person has adjusted to the new time zone. However, in some cases symptoms may persist. If symptoms are still present after more than 2 weeks, then patients should be reassessed for other sleep disorders such as psychophysiologic insomnia, particularly if associated with poor sleep habits, or for continued circadian misalignment owing to antidromic reentrainment. Antidromic reentrainment occurs when the circadian clock phase shifts in the opposite direction to the shift in the environment and as such the clock has further to adjust to become realigned. For example, when traveling east the goal is to phase advance, if the clock instead phase delays this would be antidromic reentrainment. Exceptions to this are when a very large phase advance is required (~11 + hours) after travel east, in this case it may take less time to reentrain with a phase delay. Finally, if gastrointestinal or other physical complaints persist, then the patient should be reassessed for other underlying medical conditions.[9,10]

SHIFT WORK DISORDER

Shift work is typically defined as work outside of the hours of 6 AM through 8 PM. Although about 20% of the workers in most industrialized countries are employed in some form of shift work,[39] it is estimated that only 5% to 10% of these workers have shift work disorder.[40] A summary of the symptoms, diagnosis and treatment of shift work disorder is provided in **Table 2**. Shift work disorder is characterized by symptoms of insomnia and/or excessive sleepiness associated with the shift work schedule. It is diagnosed by history, but the use of sleep and work logs either alone or in combination with wrist actigraphy for either 2 weeks or for the duration of the shift rotation can be useful.[9,10] An example of a wrist activity record for a night shift worker (work between 11 PM and 7 AM) is provided in **Fig. 2**; this figure also demonstrates the timing of several therapeutic interventions.

Not all shift workers have shift work disorder and some recent evidence suggests that there are physiologic differences in those with shift work disorder compared with shift workers without the disorder. For example, those with shift work disorder have shorter sleep duration, shorter sleep latency on the multiple sleep latency test, hyperreactivity to novel stimuli, and reduced brain response to auditory stimuli as measured by brain event-related potentials.[41–43] It has also been suggested that there are 2 distinct phenotypes within those with shift work disorder, namely, those with insomnia and sleepiness and those with only insomnia. Patients with both insomnia and sleepiness were found to be more likely to have a long tandem repeat on PER3 than those with insomnia but no sleepiness.[44] Similar polymorphisms in PER3 have been shown by others to be more common in those with an evening chronotype and

delayed sleep–wake phase disorder and to be associated with alterations in performance and sleep homeostasis.[45–49] Given the number and type of differences between shift workers with and without shift work disorder, it is not unreasonable to propose that those with the disorder may be at a greater risk for adverse outcomes related to shift work.

Factors that may predispose people to poor adaptation to shift work include the type of shift schedule, age, gender, and chronotype.[50–53] Shift work may also exacerbate preexisting psychiatric disorders that are susceptible to sleep loss and circadian misalignment, including depression, bipolar depression, and substance abuse.[10,54] Chronotype is a person's preference for being active and alert at a particular time of day (ie, morning lark or evening owl) and is thought to have a biological and genetic basis.[45,46] It has been measured in various ways, including questionnaires about a person's preference to conduct various activities at a particular time of day[55] or by determining typical sleep times.[56] Having an evening chronotype is thought to aid in adjustment to shift work. However, it is not always feasible for a worker to work in a profession/schedule that is in line with their chronotype and there are often other factors that interact to further impact sleep. In a recent study of nurses in the intensive care unit in which the majority where morning chronotypes (64%), compared with evening types, the morning type nurses were more likely to nap before the night shifts, which is considered a good strategy to reduce homeostatic sleep load before work, and to have young children at home, which is often associated with short sleep in shift workers.[57] Evening chronotype and sleep disturbance are both associated with depressive symptoms, and in shift workers sleep disturbance is prevalent. Lee and colleagues[58] examined the complex interactions between chronotype, insomnia, and emotional disturbance. In a study of nurses on a shift work schedule, they showed that sleep disturbance is prevalent (70%) and that this is mediated by emotional disturbance and insomnia vulnerability, but not chronotype. Lee and coworkers[59] have also shown that nurses working shift work are at a 1.5 times increased likelihood of having greater symptoms of depression.

Competing demands on a person's time between shifts also contribute to how a person copes with shift work, and can impact the amount of time that is dedicated to sleep.[52,60] Women often assume the bulk of the domestic work responsibilities, and for many women shift work can be an additional burden that is associated with poor

Table 2
Summary of the symptoms, diagnosis and treatment of jet lag disorder

Symptoms	Diagnosis	Treatment		
		Direction of Travel	Time of Intervention	Intervention
• Insomnia • Excessive sleepiness • Malaise • Gastrointestinal disturbance • Decreased performance	• History • Travel across ≥2 times zones	East	Before travel	Phase advance Three days before travel • Start to move sleep period 1 h earlier each day • Bright light (1 h) upon waking in morning • Melatonin 5 h before usual bedtime
			Destination	• Minimize morning light (sunglasses, remain indoors) • Maximize afternoon light (go outside or light box) • Hypnotics at bedtime - zolpidem 10 mg, up to 3 nights • Melatonin (2–5 mg) before bedtime, repeat up to 4 nights • Short nap (<30 min) • Sleep hygiene
		West	Before travel/ destination	Phase delay • Minimize early morning light (sun glasses, remain indoors) • Maximize evening light (go outside or light box) • Hypnotics at bedtime - zolpidem 10 mg, up to 3 nights • Caffeine, but avoid close to bedtime • Short nap (<30 min) • Sleep hygiene

mental health outcomes.[61] Stress is another factor that can impact both sleep and cardiovascular health. There is evidence that work-related stressors may be greater for some shift workers compared with day workers. For example, working night or afternoon shifts was associated with greater total stress in police officers, even after controlling for age, sex, rank, and race/ethnicity.[62]

Shift work itself is associated with numerous poor health outcomes similar to those seen with sleep loss and circadian misalignment, such as diabetes, obesity, hypertension, impaired reproductive health, cognitive function, and cancer.[40,61,63–66] It is likely that duration of shift work exposure, the number of night shifts worked per month, and the age at which a person started shift work also play a role in the development of poor health outcomes. For example, shift work is associated with poor cognitive function that is related to the duration of shift work exposure particularly when exposure was more than 10 years. The

good news is that it seems that the effects of shift work on cognition are potentially reversible after at least 5 years of no longer working a shift work schedule.[67] Nurses who work more than 8 night shifts per month are 3.9 times more likely to be obese.[65] Using the Nurses' Health Study II, Ramin and colleagues[68] found that ever working shift work was associated with obesity, greater caloric intake, and short sleep duration. These associations were impacted by age at which shift work was performed and if shift work was performed before age 25 this was associated with fewer risk factors than shift work later in life. In addition to higher caloric intake, shift workers are also likely to have alterations in food preference. Cain and colleagues[69] recently reported a greater preference for high-fat foods after a simulated night shift schedule.

There is also evidence that shift work may worsen sleep apnea. In a study where the apnea hypopnea index was assessed both during day sleep and night sleep in shift workers, the apnea

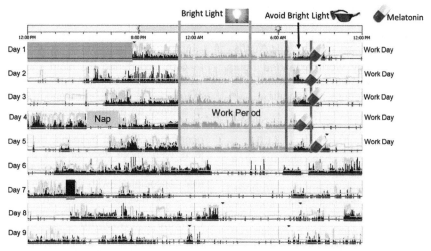

Fig. 2. Wrist activity recording from a night shift worker with shift work disorder. Each line represents 24 hours (12 PM–12 PM). This person worked 5 consecutive night shifts between 11 PM and 7 AM (*light green*), and was in bed between 8:30 and 9:00 AM after their shifts, whereas they went to bed between 10 PM and 1 AM on their days off (days 6–9). On day 3, the patient had a very short sleep period, so on day 4 they supplemented their main sleep period with a nap (indicated in *orange*). In this scenario, the patient should seek bright light between 11 PM and 4 AM (indicated by *blue box*), but avoid light between 6:30 AM and 8:30 AM (indicated by *red bars*). They could also take melatonin before daytime sleep (indicated by *red* and *white capsule*). Black bars indicate activity and yellow lines indicate light exposure; blue bars indicate off-wrist, gray bars indicate the time before recording started, and blue triangles indicate when the patient pushed an event marker to indicate bed or wake time.

hypopnea index was higher during the day time sleep periods.[70] Because apnea events are more likely to occur during rapid eye movement (REM) sleep, the higher apnea hypopnea index during day sleep is potentially owing to the circadian rhythm in REM sleep. REM sleep occurs more in the biological morning, regardless of prior wakefulness.[71] This has implications for treatment of other sleep disorders in shift workers.

A multimodal approach is recommended when addressing the symptoms of insomnia and excessive sleepiness associated with shift work disorder. Although various interventions have been tested to reduce the negative impact of shift work on sleep and wakefulness and to improve circadian alignment (see **Table 2**), many of these interventions have only been tested during simulated night shift schedules in nonshift workers. There is a need for further studies to examine the impact of these interventions in shift workers and those with shift work disorder. Despite these limitations, the strategies discussed herein are currently considered the standard of care for the treatment of shift work disorder by the American Academy of Sleep Medicine.[20] It is yet to be determined whether these interventions impact the long-term health of shift workers.[64] However, regardless of the long-term implications, these interventions do immediately impact sleep and quality of life in shift workers.

Sleep Hygiene

Maintaining good sleep hygiene practices is a central component of the treatment of shift work disorder. Maintaining regular sleep–wake times, when the work schedule allows, that permit an adequate amount of time in bed each day is important. Furthermore, because shift work may be associated with a more stressful work environment,[62] it is important to allow for an adequate time to relax before bedtime. It is also important to keep the sleeping environment cool, dark, and quiet, which can be a challenge when trying to sleep during the daytime.

Circadian Realignment

Aligning the timing of endogenous circadian rhythms with the altered sleep–wake and work schedule may improve sleep and reduce excessive sleepiness. Realignment is typically achieved by a combination of appropriately timed light/dark exposure and/or administration of melatonin.[72–79] However, this approach can be challenging owing to social factors that compete with the required changes to the light/dark and sleep/wake schedule. Depending on the type of shift work schedule, circadian alignment may not be advisable and in these cases direct symptomatic treatment may be more appropriate. For example, some individuals may only work a single night shift each week or may work extended hours that include night work, such as physicians, firefighters, and other emergency personnel.

Bright Light

Bright light exposure can be used acutely to improve alertness and/or to phase shift the circadian clock. Several studies have shown that bright light (3000–5000 lux), even intermittently applied during the first half of the night shift, improves alertness immediately, and over time speed the alignment of the sleep–wake and circadian systems.[72–79] To maintain this alignment, shift workers are also instructed to avoid bright light by using dark glasses in the morning on the way home from work or while outdoors.[75,79]

Melatonin Administration

Melatonin for the treatment of shift work disorder has varied results depending on the time of administration. The usual recommendation is to take melatonin before the daytime sleep period owing to the hypnotic effects at this time, resulting in improved sleep.[80–82] Although melatonin at sleep onset will also likely phase delay the clock, if the patient does not avoid bright light in the morning, any phase shifting benefits of melatonin at this time may be counteracted, because light is a stronger entraining agent for the circadian clock than melatonin.[75]

Compromise Phase Position

For shift workers who only have a few days off in between consecutive night shifts, it might be beneficial to try and maintain their work-day sleep–wake schedule during their days off. In other words, they would continue to sleep during the day and be awake at night. However, this is not always possible for most workers. An alternative is to try and keep what has been termed a compromise phase position. Benefits to sleep, performance, and well-being have been demonstrated in a series of publications of data from a simulated night shift schedule where such a compromise phase position was maintained, in combination with interventions to speed the alignment of the circadian clock to the night work schedule.[83–85] In this series of studies, the night shift was between 11 PM and 7 AM and the sleep time on work days was between about 8 AM to 4 PM. On nonwork days, the subjects kept a sleep–wake schedule that was a compromise between their normal nocturnal sleep time and the sleep time on work days. In this case sleep times were between 3 AM and 12 AM In addition to the altered sleep–wake schedule they were given intermittent bright light (~4100 lux) during the night shift and asked to wear dark glasses when outside, especially in the morning. Using this intervention, they were able to achieve an average dim light melatonin onset of 4:34 AM compared with a dim light melatonin onset of 9:00 PM at baseline, indicating that subjects were more appropriately aligned with their new work schedule. The improved alignment was also associated with improvements in performance on a simple reaction time task.

Caffeine and Napping

For shift workers, strategic use of caffeine or naps individually can both be beneficial in improving alertness; however, the benefits are increased when used in combination.[86] The amount of caffeine required depends on individual tolerance, but should be avoided for at least a few hours before bedtime. Napping can be used as a way to supplement the daytime sleep period and, as such, naps before starting work will aid in dissipating the homeostatic need for sleep. In this case, naps can be of a longer duration depending on the duration of the prior sleep period. When possible and if necessary, napping while at work for even a short period of time (as little as 10 minutes) can improve performance for several hours.[87–89] However, napping is not a replacement for good daytime sleep. When using caffeine and napping in combination[89] to improve alertness, it is recommended to take the caffeine before a 30-minute nap, because it takes approximately 30 minutes for the alerting benefits of caffeine to take effect.

Hypnotics

Short-acting hypnotics such as zolpidem can be used to treat insomnia associated with the daytime sleep period in shift workers.[90–92] However, there is a need to monitor use and multiple prescriptions for different agents in shift workers. A recent study in nurses working shift work schedules suggests that the use of multiple hypnotics is associated with greater depressive symptoms, worse quality of life, and work performance than single hypnotic users.[93] Although this association is not necessarily unique to shift workers, it does highlight the importance of monitoring for polypharmacy.

Modafinil and Armodafinil

Both modafinil and armodafinil are approved by the US Food and Drug Administration (FDA) for the treatment of hypersomnia associated with shift work disorder. Typically, modafinil (200 mg) or armodafinil (150 mg) are administered at the beginning of the shift. If necessary, the dose can be increased to optimize alertness. Because the improvements in sleepiness are generally small,[94–96] it is important that patients be aware of the signs of excessive sleepiness and fatigue and the potential of increased risk of sleepiness-related accidents. Drake and colleagues[97] recently conducted a study in night shift workers to examine whether 150 mg of armodafinil or placebo given at 11:45 PM (on average 3.25 hours after the average reported shift start time) would improve alertness and performance on a simulated driving task, with particular focus on the time of a typical commute home after a night shift. Although this study showed that armodafinil reduced weaving and off-road deviations at 7 AM and 9 AM, there was still excessive sleepiness at 7 AM and 7:30 AM, as indicated by an average sleep latency of about 7 minutes, and an average of more than 5 off-road events.

CONSIDERATIONS WHEN USING BRIGHT LIGHT OR EXOGENOUS MELATONIN

When using timed bright light and melatonin as interventions to treat the symptoms of jet lag and shift work disorder, there are several factors to consider. In addition to its effects on the circadian clock bright light also has direct alerting effects,[98,99] which may be important to improve alertness in someone who is sleepy owing to jet lag or shift work disorder. Therefore, although avoiding light at certain times of day is recommended to avoid shifting the circadian clock in the wrong direction, if the individual is already sleepy avoidance of bright light could further exacerbate this. If a shift worker has excessive sleepiness in the early morning (when it is recommended to avoid bright light), an alternate means of transportation home (public transportation, or employer-paid vouchers for private transportation [eg, taxis]) should be considered when possible. Another consideration is that bright light may exacerbate migraines,[100] so other interventions may need to be used in those with a history of migraines.

Melatonin is not regulated by the FDA, so it is not approved for use in either jet lag or shift work disorder. The recommendations presented in this article are based on research studies supporting the use of melatonin to phase shift the circadian clock. The exact dose of melatonin to take has not been determined adequately for jet lag or shift work disorder, but experimental studies suggest that 5 mg or less is usually adequate.[20] Owing to the hypnotic effects of melatonin taken during the "biological day," administration at this time may result in excessive sleepiness, particularly at higher doses,[31,101] and caution should be used if driving. In addition, pregnant women are advised not to take melatonin.

DISCUSSION

There will always be a need for work schedules that cover every hour of the day. Although we know that working against our endogenous circadian clock has a significant negative impact on sleep, health, performance, and safety, there are limited studies in "real-life" settings regarding effectiveness and practical implementation of the currently recommended treatments. Future research is needed to develop practical interventions and/or schedules that limit the negative impact of shift work on health, performance, and safety. For example, an area requiring further investigation is the development and testing of new technologies to monitor sleepiness, sleep, activity level, and caloric intake in shift workers. New personal health devices such as Fitbit and Jawbone allow people to monitor their sleep, caloric intake, and activity level. The recommendations these devices provide about behavioral change would likely benefit from further validation for people who do shift work. An additional challenge is the issue of chronic sleep loss, in that individuals are often not very good at self-assessing alertness or their level of performance impairment.[102,103] One technique that has been used widely to monitor alertness objectively is the measurement of eye movements. In a recent study, the use of ocular measures with a new device was predictive of sleepiness and circadian alignment in simulated shift work.[104] These devices could be another tool to measure the impact of new interventions on waking function.

For some people, frequent travel across multiple times zones is required for work, and it is unclear what the health impact is of repeated long-term exposure to jet lag. The consequences are likely to be similar to that seen with shift work. For example, international airline pilots and flight crew perform both shift work and travel across multiple time zones, and although work hours in the airline industry are highly regulated to maintain safety, there remain long-term health risks associated with sleep loss and circadian misalignment to consider.

A new and potentially controversial take on shift work disorder is that the treatments for shift work disorder involve making the worker change their behavior to manage the schedule. Although the need for such treatments is unlikely to go away, on a societal level there is the opportunity to design, test, and advocate for new work schedules that limit sleep loss and circadian disruption, and yet still meet the operational needs of an organization. For example, there may be optimal shift start times and shift durations that are better than others. Some recent laboratory studies have examined the impact of split work/sleep schedules (2 equal work periods per 24 hours), that are common in the maritime industry,[105] on sleep and performance, and indicate that both sleep and performance may be better compared with a single night shift.[106] This is thought to be owing to the ability of the person to dissipate their homeostatic sleep load, which builds up the longer they are awake, with 2 sleep periods per day rather than a single consolidated sleep period.

Given the adverse consequences on physical, mental, and cognitive health of both short-term and chronic circadian misalignment, more research is need to inform the development of guidelines for optimizing the health of those who need to be awake during the night or early morning hours.

REFERENCES

1. Wever R. The circadian system of man. New York: Springer-Verlag; 1979.
2. Klein DC, Moore RY, Reppert SM. Suprachiasmatic nucleus - the mind's clock. New York: Oxford University Press; 1991. p. 467.
3. Bass J. Circadian topology of metabolism. Nature 2012;491(7424):348–56.
4. Dibner C, Schibler U, Albrecht U. The mammalian circadian timing system: organization and coordination of central and peripheral clocks. Annu Rev Physiol 2010;72:517–49.
5. Czeisler CA, Duffy JF, Shanahan TL, et al. Stability, precision, and near-24-hour period of the human circadian pacemaker. Science 1999;284(5423): 2177–81.
6. Aschoff J, Fatranska M, Giedke H, et al. Human circadian rhythms in continuous darkness: entrainment by social cues. Science 1971;171:213–5.
7. Mills JN, Minors DS, Waterhouse JM. The circadian rhythms of human subjects without timepieces or indication of the alternation of day and night. J Physiol 1974;240(3):567–94.
8. Zelinski EL, Deibel SH, McDonald RJ. The trouble with circadian clock dysfunction: multiple deleterious effects on the brain and body. Neurosci Biobehav Rev 2014;40:80–101.
9. American Psychiatric Association, DSM-5 Task Force. Diagnostic and statistical manual of mental disorders:

DSM-5. 5th edition. Washington, DC: American Psychiatric Association; 2013. p. xliv. p. 947.
10. ICSD-3. The international classification of sleep disorders: diagnostic and coding manual. 2nd edition. Darien (IL): American Academy of Sleep Medicine; 2014.
11. Khalsa SB, Jewett ME, Cajochen C, et al. A phase response curve to single bright light pulses in human subjects. J Physiol 2003;549(Pt 3):945–52.
12. Minors DS, Waterhouse JM, Wirz-Justice A. A human phase-response curve to light. Neurosci Lett 1991; 133(1):36–40.
13. Wright HR, Lack LC. Effect of light wavelength on suppression and phase delay of the melatonin rhythm. Chronobiol Int 2001;18(5):801–8.
14. Lockley SW, Brainard GC, Czeisler CA. High sensitivity of the human circadian melatonin rhythm to resetting by short wavelength light. J Clin Endocrinol Metab 2003;88(9):4502–5.
15. Kim SJ, Benloucif S, Reid KJ, et al. Phase-shifting response to light in older adults. J Physiol 2014; 592(Pt 1):189–202.
16. Dewan K, Benloucif S, Reid K, et al. Light-induced changes of the circadian clock of humans: increasing duration is more effective than increasing light intensity. Sleep 2011;34(5): 593–9.
17. Burgess HJ, Revell VL, Eastman CI. A three pulse phase response curve to three milligrams of melatonin in humans. J Physiol 2008;586(2):639–47.
18. Lewy AL, Ahmed S, Jackson JML, et al. Melatonin shifts human circadian rhythms according to a phase-response curve. Chronobiol Int 1992;9: 380–92.
19. Burgess HJ, Revell VL, Molina TA, et al. Human phase response curves to three days of daily melatonin: 0.5 mg versus 3.0 mg. J Clin Endocrinol Metab 2010;95(7):3325–31.
20. Morgenthaler TI, Lee-Chiong T, Alessi C, et al. Practice parameters for the clinical evaluation and treatment of circadian rhythm sleep disorders. An American Academy of Sleep Medicine report. Sleep 2007;30(11):1445–59.
21. Administration IT. U.S. citizen traffic to overseas regions, Canada & Mexico 2014. In: Commerce OO, editor. Washington, DC: Office of Travel and Tourism Industries; 2014. Available at: http://travel.trade.gov/view/m-2014-O-001/index.html. Accessed August 2, 2015.
22. Leger D. The prevalence of jet-lag among 507 traveling businessmen. Sleep Res 1993;22:409.
23. Burgess HJ, Crowley SJ, Gazda CJ, et al. Preflight adjustment to eastward travel: 3 days of advancing sleep with and without morning bright light. J Biol Rhythms 2003;18(4):318–28.
24. Revell VL, Burgess HJ, Gazda CJ, et al. Advancing human circadian rhythms with afternoon melatonin

and morning intermittent bright light. J Clin Endocrinol Metab 2006;91(1):54–9.

25. Crowley SJ, Eastman CI. Phase advancing human circadian rhythms with morning bright light, afternoon melatonin, and gradually shifted sleep: can we reduce morning bright-light duration? Sleep Med 2015;16(2):288–97.

26. Boulos Z, Campbell SS, Lewy AJ, et al. Light treatment for sleep disorders: consensus report. VII. Jet lag. J Biol Rhythms 1995;10(2):167–76.

27. Daan S, Lewy AJ. Scheduled exposure to daylight: a potential strategy to reduce "jet lag" following transmeridian flight. Psychopharmacol Bull 1984; 20(3):566–8.

28. Waterhouse J, Reilly T, Atkinson G. Jet-lag. Lancet 1997;350(9091):1611–6.

29. Edwards BJ, Atkinson G, Waterhouse J, et al. Use of melatonin in recovery from jet-lag following an eastward flight across 10 time-zones. Ergonomics 2000;43(10):1501–13.

30. Herxheimer A, Petrie KJ. Melatonin for the prevention and treatment of jetlag. Cochrane Database Syst Rev 2003;(1):CD001520.

31. Wyatt JK, Dijk DJ, Ritz-de Cecco A, et al. Sleep-facilitating effect of exogenous melatonin in healthy young men and women is circadian-phase dependent. Sleep 2006;29(5):609–18.

32. Suhner A, Schlagenhauf P, Hofer I, et al. Effectiveness and tolerability of melatonin and zolpidem for the alleviation of jet lag. Aviat Space Environ Med 2001;72(7):638–46.

33. Jamieson AO, Zammit GK, Rosenberg RS, et al. Zolpidem reduces the sleep disturbance of jet lag. Sleep Med 2001;2(5):423–30.

34. Zee PC, Wang-Weigand S, Wright KP Jr, et al. Effects of ramelteon on insomnia symptoms induced by rapid, eastward travel. Sleep Med 2010;11(6):525–33.

35. Canton JL, Smith MR, Choi HS, et al. Phase delaying the human circadian clock with a single light pulse and moderate delay of the sleep/dark episode: no influence of iris color. J Circadian Rhythms 2009;7:8.

36. Smith MR, Eastman CI. Phase delaying the human circadian clock with blue-enriched polychromatic light. Chronobiol Int 2009;26(4):709–25.

37. Petrie K, Conaglen JV, Thompson L, et al. Effect of melatonin on jet lag after long haul flights. BMJ 1989;298(6675):705–7.

38. Petrie K, Dawson AG, Thompson L, et al. A double-blind trial of melatonin as a treatment for jet lag in international cabin crew. Biol Psychiatry 1993; 33(7):526–30.

39. US Department of Labor, Bureau of Labor Statistics. Workers on flexible and shift schedules in 2004 summary. 2004. Available at: http://www.bls.gov/news.release/flex.nr0.htm. Accessed August 2, 2015.

40. Drake CL, Roehrs T, Richardson G, et al. Shift work sleep disorder: prevalence and consequences beyond that of symptomatic day workers. Sleep 2004;27(8):1453–62.

41. Gumenyuk V, Howard R, Roth T, et al. Sleep loss, circadian mismatch, and abnormalities in reorienting of attention in night workers with shift work disorder. Sleep 2014;37(3):545–56.

42. Gumenyuk V, Roth T, Drake CL. Circadian phase, sleepiness, and light exposure assessment in night workers with and without shift work disorder. Chronobiol Int 2012;29(7):928–36.

43. Gumenyuk V, Roth T, Korzyukov O, et al. Shift work sleep disorder is associated with an attenuated brain response of sensory memory and an increased brain response to novelty: an ERP study. Sleep 2010;33(5):703–13.

44. Gumenyuk V, Belcher R, Drake CL, et al. Differential sleep, sleepiness, and neurophysiology in the insomnia phenotypes of shift work disorder. Sleep 2015;38(1):119–26.

45. Archer SN, Carpen JD, Gibson M, et al. Polymorphism in the PER3 promoter associates with diurnal preference and delayed sleep phase disorder. Sleep 2010;33(5):695–701.

46. Archer SN, Robilliard DL, Skene DJ, et al. A length polymorphism in the circadian clock gene Per3 is linked to delayed sleep phase syndrome and extreme diurnal preference. Sleep 2003;26(4): 413–5.

47. Ebisawa T, Uchiyama M, Kajimura N, et al. Association of structural polymorphisms in the human period3 gene with delayed sleep phase syndrome. EMBO Rep 2001;2(4):342–6.

48. Goel N, Banks S, Mignot E, et al. PER3 polymorphism predicts cumulative sleep homeostatic but not neurobehavioral changes to chronic partial sleep deprivation. PLoS One 2009;4(6):e5874.

49. Viola AU, Archer SN, James LM, et al. PER3 polymorphism predicts sleep structure and waking performance. Curr Biol 2007;17(7):613–8.

50. Folkard S, Monk TH, Lobban MC. Short and long-term adjustment of circadian rhythms in 'permanent' night nurses. Ergonomics 1978;21(10):785–99.

51. Harma MI, Hakola T, Akerstedt T, et al. Age and adjustment to night work. Occup Environ Med 1994;51(8):568–73.

52. Presser H. Working in a 24/7 economy: challenges for American families. New York: Russell Sage Foundation; 2003.

53. Smith L, Mason C. Age and the subjective experience of shiftwork. J Hum Ergol 2001;30(1–2):307–13.

54. Meyrer R, Demling J, Kornhuber J, et al. Effects of night shifts in bipolar disorders and extreme morningness. Bipolar Disord 2009;11(8):897–9.

55. Horne JA, Ostberg O. A self-assessment questionnaire to determine morningness-eveningness in human circadian rhythms. Int J Chronobiol 1976; 4(2):97–110.

56. Juda M, Vetter C, Roenneberg T. The Munich chronotype questionnaire for shift-workers (MCTQShift). J Biol Rhythms 2013;28(2):130–40.

57. Reinke L, Ozbay Y, Dieperink W, et al. The effect of chronotype on sleepiness, fatigue, and psychomotor vigilance of ICU nurses during the night shift. Intensive Care Med 2015;41(4):657–66.

58. Lee CY, Chen HC, Meg Tseng MC, et al. The relationships among sleep quality and chronotype, emotional disturbance, and insomnia vulnerability in shift nurses. J Nurs Res 2015;23(3):225–35.

59. Lee HY, Kim MS, Kim O, et al. Association between shift work and severity of depressive symptoms among female nurses: the Korea nurses' health study. J Nurs Manag 2015. [Epub ahead of print].

60. White L, Keith B. The effect of shift work on the quality and stability of marital relations. J Marriage Fam 1990;52(2):453–62.

61. Rotenberg L, Silva-Costa A, Griep RH. Mental health and poor recovery in female nursing workers: a contribution to the study of gender inequities. Rev Panam Salud Publica 2014;35(3):179–85.

62. Ma CC, Andrew ME, Fekedulegn D, et al. Shift work and occupational stress in police officers. Saf Health Work 2015;6(1):25–9.

63. Brum MC, Filho FF, Schnorr CC, et al. Shift work and its association with metabolic disorders. Diabetol Metab Syndr 2015;7:45.

64. Neil-Sztramko SE, Pahwa M, Demers PA, et al. Health-related interventions among night shift workers: a critical review of the literature. Scand J Work Environ Health 2014;40(6):543–56.

65. Peplonska B, Bukowska A, Sobala W. Association of rotating night shift work with BMI and abdominal obesity among nurses and midwives. PLoS One 2015;10(7):e0133761.

66. He C, Anand ST, Ebell MH, et al. Circadian disrupting exposures and breast cancer risk: a meta-analysis. Int Arch Occup Environ Health 2015;88(5):533–47.

67. Marquie JC, Tucker P, Folkard S, et al. Chronic effects of shift work on cognition: findings from the VISAT longitudinal study. Occup Environ Med 2015;72(4):258–64.

68. Ramin C, Devore EE, Wang W, et al. Night shift work at specific age ranges and chronic disease risk factors. Occup Environ Med 2015;72(2):100–7.

69. Cain SW, Filtness AJ, Phillips CL, et al. Enhanced preference for high-fat foods following a simulated night shift. Scand J Work Environ Health 2015; 41(3):288–93.

70. Paciorek M, Korczynski P, Bielicki P, et al. Obstructive sleep apnea in shift workers. Sleep Med 2011; 12(3):274–7.

71. Dijk DJ, Czeisler CA. Contribution of the circadian pacemaker and the sleep homeostat to sleep propensity, sleep structure, electroencephalographic slow waves, and sleep spindle activity in humans. J Neurosci 1995;15(5 Pt 1):3526–38.

72. Boivin DB, James FO. Circadian adaptation to night-shift work by judicious light and darkness exposure. J Biol Rhythms 2002;17(6):556–67.

73. Burgess HJ, Sharkey KM, Eastman CI. Bright light, dark and melatonin can promote circadian adaptation in night shift workers. Sleep Med Rev 2002; 6(5):407–20.

74. Campbell SS, Dijk DJ, Boulos Z, et al. Light treatment for sleep disorders: consensus report. III. Alerting and activating effects. J Biol Rhythms 1995;10(2):129–32.

75. Crowley SJ, Lee C, Tseng CY, et al. Combinations of bright light, scheduled dark, sunglasses, and melatonin to facilitate circadian entrainment to night shift work. J Biol Rhythms 2003;18(6):513–23.

76. Dawson D, Campbell SS. Timed exposure to bright light improves sleep and alertness during simulated night shifts. Sleep 1991;14(6):511–6.

77. Dawson D, Encel N, Lushington K. Improving adaptation to simulated night shift: timed exposure to bright light versus daytime melatonin administration. Sleep 1995;18(1):11–21.

78. Eastman CI, Liu L, Fogg LF. Circadian rhythm adaptation to simulated night shift work: effect of nocturnal bright-light duration. Sleep 1995;18(6):399–407.

79. Eastman CI, Stewart KT, Mahoney MP, et al. Dark goggles and bright light improve circadian rhythm adaptation to night-shift work. Sleep 1994;17(6):535–43.

80. Sharkey KM, Eastman CI. Melatonin phase shifts human circadian rhythms in a placebo-controlled simulated night-work study. Am J Physiol Regul Integr Comp Physiol 2002;282(2):R454–63.

81. Sharkey KM, Fogg LF, Eastman CI. Effects of melatonin administration on daytime sleep after simulated night shift work. J Sleep Res 2001;10(3):181–92.

82. Smith MR, Lee C, Crowley SJ, et al. Morning melatonin has limited benefit as a soporific for daytime sleep after night work. Chronobiol Int 2005;22(5):873–88.

83. Smith MR, Cullnan EE, Eastman CI. Shaping the light/dark pattern for circadian adaptation to night shift work. Physiol Behav 2008;95(3):449–56.

84. Smith MR, Fogg LF, Eastman CI. A compromise circadian phase position for permanent night work improves mood, fatigue, and performance. Sleep 2009;32(11):1481–9.

85. Smith MR, Fogg LF, Eastman CI. Practical interventions to promote circadian adaptation to permanent night shift work: study 4. J Biol Rhythms 2009; 24(2):161–72.

86. Ker K, Edwards PJ, Felix LM, et al. Caffeine for the prevention of injuries and errors in shift workers. Cochrane Database Syst Rev 2010;(5):CD008508.

87. Purnell MT, Feyer AM, Herbison GP. The impact of a nap opportunity during the night shift on the performance and alertness of 12-h shift workers. J Sleep Res 2002;11(3):219–27.

88. Sallinen M, Harma M, Akerstedt T, et al. Promoting alertness with a short nap during a night shift. J Sleep Res 1998;7(4):240–7.

89. Schweitzer PK, Randazzo AC, Stone K, et al. Laboratory and field studies of naps and caffeine as practical countermeasures for sleep-wake problems associated with night work. Sleep 2006;29(1):39–50.

90. Hart CL, Ward AS, Haney M, et al. Zolpidem-related effects on performance and mood during simulated night-shift work. Exp Clin Psychopharmacol 2003;11(4):259–68.

91. Walsh JK, Schweitzer PK, Anch AM, et al. Sleepiness/alertness on a simulated night shift following sleep at home with triazolam. Sleep 1991;14(2):140–6.

92. Walsh JK, Sugerman JL, Muehlbach MJ, et al. Physiological sleep tendency on a simulated night shift: adaptation and effects of triazolam. Sleep 1988;11(3):251–64.

93. Futenma K, Asaoka S, Takaesu Y, et al. Impact of hypnotics use on daytime function and factors associated with usage by female shift work nurses. Sleep Med 2015;16(5):604–11.

94. Czeisler CA, Walsh JK, Roth T, et al. Modafinil for excessive sleepiness associated with shift-work sleep disorder. N Engl J Med 2005;353(5):476–86.

95. Czeisler CA, Walsh JK, Wesnes KA, et al. Armodafinil for treatment of excessive sleepiness associated with shift work disorder: a randomized controlled study. Mayo Clin Proc 2009;84(11):958–72.

96. Erman MK, Rosenberg R, Modafinil Shift Work Sleep Disorder Study Group. Modafinil for excessive sleepiness associated with chronic shift work sleep disorder: effects on patient functioning and health-related quality of life. Prim Care Companion J Clin Psychiatry 2007;9(3):188–94.

97. Drake C, Gumenyuk V, Roth T, et al. Effects of armodafinil on simulated driving and alertness in shift work disorder. Sleep 2014;37(12):1987–94.

98. Cajochen C, Zeitzer JM, Czeisler CA, et al. Dose-response relationship for light intensity and ocular and electroencephalographic correlates of human alertness. Behav Brain Res 2000;115(1):75–83.

99. Cajochen C. Alerting effects of light. Sleep Med Rev 2007;11(6):453–64.

100. Ulrich V, Olesen J, Gervil M, et al. Possible risk factors and precipitants for migraine with aura in discordant twin-pairs: a population-based study. Cephalalgia 2000;20(9):821–5.

101. Reid K, Van den Heuvel C, Dawson D. Day-time melatonin administration: effects on core temperature and sleep onset latency. J Sleep Res 1996;5(3):150–4.

102. Biggs SN, Smith A, Dorrian J, et al. Perception of simulated driving performance after sleep restriction and caffeine. J Psychosom Res 2007;63(6):573–7.

103. Dorrian J, Lamond N, Dawson D. The ability to self-monitor performance when fatigued. J Sleep Res 2000;9(2):137–44.

104. Ftouni S, Sletten TL, Nicholas CL, et al. Ocular measures of sleepiness are increased in night shift workers undergoing a simulated night shift near the peak time of the 6-sulfatoxymelatonin rhythm. J Clin Sleep Med 2015. [Epub ahead of print].

105. Short MA, Agostini A, Lushington K, et al. A systematic review of the sleep, sleepiness, and performance implications of limited wake shift work schedules. Scand J Work Environ Health 2015;41(5):425–40.

106. Jackson ML, Banks S, Belenky G. Investigation of the effectiveness of a split sleep schedule in sustaining sleep and maintaining performance. Chronobiol Int 2014;31(10):1218–30.

United States Postal Service

Statement of Ownership, Management, and Circulation
(All Periodicals Publications Except Requestor Publications)

1. Publication Title	2. Publication Number	3. Filing Date
Sleep Medicine Clinics	0 2 5 – 0 5 3	9/18/15

4. Issue Frequency	5. Number of Issues Published Annually	6. Annual Subscription Price
Mar, Jun, Sep, Dec	4	$195.00

7. Complete Mailing Address of Known Office of Publication *(Not printer)(Street, city, county, state, and ZIP+4®)*

Elsevier Inc.
360 Park Avenue South
New York, NY 10010-1710

Contact Person
Stephen R. Bushing

Telephone *(Include area code)*
215-239-3688

8. Complete Mailing Address of Headquarters or General Business Office of Publisher *(Not printer)*

Elsevier Inc., 360 Park Avenue South, New York, NY 10010-1710

9. Full Names and Complete Mailing Addresses of Publisher, Editor, and Managing Editor *(Do not leave blank)*

Publisher *(Name and complete mailing address)*

Linda Belfus, Elsevier Inc., 1600 John F. Kennedy Blvd., Suite 1800, Philadelphia, PA 19103

Editor *(Name and complete mailing address)*

Patrick Manley, Elsevier Inc., 1600 John F. Kennedy Blvd., Suite 1800, Philadelphia, PA 19103-2899

Managing Editor *(Name and complete mailing address)*

Adrianne Brigido, Elsevier Inc., 1600 John F. Kennedy Blvd., Suite 1800, Philadelphia, PA 19103-2899

10. Owner *(Do not leave blank. If the publication is owned by a corporation, give the name and address of the corporation immediately followed by the names and addresses of all stockholders owning or holding 1 percent or more of the total amount of stock. If not owned by a corporation, give the names and addresses of the individual owners. If owned by a partnership or other unincorporated firm, give its name and address as well as those of each individual owner. If the publication is published by a nonprofit organization, give its name and address.)*

Full Name	Complete Mailing Address
Wholly owned subsidiary of	1600 John F. Kennedy Blvd. Ste. 1800
Reed/Elsevier, US holdings	Philadelphia, PA 19103-2899

11. Known Bondholders, Mortgagees, and Other Security Holders Owning or Holding 1 Percent or More of Total Amount of Bonds, Mortgages, or Other Securities. If none, check box ☐ None

Full Name	Complete Mailing Address
N/A	

12. Tax Status *(For completion by nonprofit organizations authorized to mail at nonprofit rates) (Check one)*
The purpose, function, and nonprofit status of this organization and the exempt status for federal income tax purposes:
☐ Has Not Changed During Preceding 12 Months
☐ Has Changed During Preceding 12 Months *(Publisher must submit explanation of change with this statement)*

PS Form 3526, July 2014 [Page 1 of 3 (Instructions Page 3)] PSN 7530-01-000-9931 **PRIVACY NOTICE:** See our Privacy policy in www.usps.com

---

13. Publication Title	14. Issue Date for Circulation Data Below
Sleep Medicine Clinics	September 2015

15. Extent and Nature of Circulation				Average No. Copies Each Issue During Preceding 12 Months	No. Copies of Single Issue Published Nearest to Filing Date
a. Total Number of Copies *(Net press run)*				481	441
b. Legitimate Paid and Or Requested Distribution (By Mail and Outside the Mail)	(1)	Mailed Outside-County Paid/Requested Mail Subscriptions stated on PS Form 3541. *(Include paid distribution above nominal rate, advertiser's proof copies and exchange copies)*		288	265
	(2)	Mailed In-County Paid/Requested Mail Subscriptions stated on PS Form 3541. *(Include paid distribution above nominal rate, advertiser's proof copies and exchange copies)*			
	(3)	Paid Distribution Outside the Mails Including Sales Through Dealers And Carriers, Street Vendors, Counter Sales, and Other Paid Distribution Outside USPS®		42	45
	(4)	Paid Distribution by Other Classes of Mail Through the USPS (e.g. First-Class Mail®)			
c. Total Paid and or Requested Circulation *(Sum of 15b (1), (2), (3), and (4))*			▶	330	310
d. Free or Nominal Rate Distribution (By Mail and Outside the Mail)	(1)	Free or Nominal Rate Outside-County Copies included on PS Form 3541		58	54
	(2)	Free or Nominal Rate In-County Copies Included on PS Form 3541			
	(3)	Free or Nominal Rate Copies mailed at Other classes Through the USPS (e.g. First-Class Mail®)			
	(4)	Free or Nominal Rate Distribution Outside the Mail (Carriers or Other means)			
e. Total Nonrequested Distribution *(Sum of 15d (1), (2), (3) and (4))*			▶	58	54
f. Total Distribution *(Sum of 15c and 15e)*			▶	388	364
g. Copies not Distributed *(See instructions to publishers #4 (page #3))*			▶	93	77
h. Total *(Sum of 15f and g)*			▶	481	441
i. Percent Paid and/or Requested Circulation *(15c divided by 15f times 100)*			▶	85.05%	85.16%

* If you are claiming electronic copies go to line 16 on page 3. If you are not claiming Electronic copies, skip to line 17 on page 3

16. Electronic Copy Circulation	Average No. Copies Each Issue During Preceding 12 Months	No. Copies of Single Issue Published Nearest to Filing Date
a. Paid Electronic Copies		
b. Total paid Print Copies *(Line 15c)* + Paid Electronic copies *(Line 16a)*		
c. Total Print Distribution *(Line 15f)* + Paid Electronic Copies *(Line 16a)*		
d. Percent Paid (Both Print & Electronic copies) *(16b divided by 16c X 100)*		

☐ I certify that 50% of all my distributed copies (electronic and print) are paid above a nominal price

17. Publication of Statement of Ownership
☐ If the publication is a general publication, publication of this statement is required. Will be printed in the **December 2015** issue of this publication.

18. Signature and Title of Editor, Publisher, Business Manager, or Owner	Date
Stephen R. Bushing	September 18, 2015
Stephen R. Bushing – Inventory Distribution Coordinator	

I certify that all information furnished on this form is true and complete. I understand that anyone who furnishes false or misleading information on this form or who omits material or information requested on the form may be subject to criminal sanctions (including fines and imprisonment) and/or civil sanctions (including civil penalties).

PS Form 3526, July 2014 (Page 3 of 3)

Moving?

Make sure your subscription moves with you!

To notify us of your new address, find your **Clinics Account Number** (located on your mailing label above your name), and contact customer service at:

Email: journalscustomerservice-usa@elsevier.com

800-654-2452 (subscribers in the U.S. & Canada)
314-447-8871 (subscribers outside of the U.S. & Canada)

Fax number: 314-447-8029

Elsevier Health Sciences Division
Subscription Customer Service
3251 Riverport Lane
Maryland Heights, MO 63043

ELSEVIER

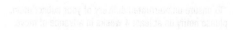

Printed and bound by CPI Group (UK) Ltd, Croydon, CR0 4YY

03/10/2024

01040381-0013